→ Bhopal %
→ Raipur
→ AFNE 2 /9
   NABL

   7pm

• Share information
• +ve -ve
• West Bengal
  SARI ?
  4K SARI Non culture
  ~ 35 - 40 ⊖ ve.
            MP / Raj
• 9-20 districts
•

~ 35 - 40 ⊖ ve.
. 9-30 District MP/Raj
.

NITRD : RK wadwa   ⑥ ✓

Gene expert ____   Blue ⎡ 8 ⎤
                   Oreen ⎣ 20 ⎦

→ Delhe / Bidar 3/7
. NABL chairman.
→ chandigarh 29/31
→ Bhopal 6/18 III
→ Raipur 8/8 ⎧ Iterklow:
              ⎩ Cratow ✓
→ AFNE 2+2 /9
    NABL

GOING VIRAL

Professor Balram Bhargava is presently the director general of the Indian Council of Medical Research (ICMR) and continues to be professor of cardiology at the All India Institute of Medical Sciences (AIIMS), New Delhi. He graduated in medicine (MBBS), followed by MD and DM, with specialization in cardiology from King George's Medical University, Lucknow. He is a fellow of the National Academy of Sciences, India (FNASc), the Indian National Science Academy (FNA), the Indian Academy of Sciences (FASc) and the National Academy of Medical Sciences India (FAMS).

He has published many research papers in national and international journals. He has been awarded the S.N. Bose Centenary award by the Indian National Science Congress, the National Academy of Sciences Platinum Jubilee Award, the Tata Innovation Fellowship, the Ranbaxy Award, the O.P. Bhasin Award, the Vasvik Award for Biomedical Technology Innovation and more recently, the UNESCO Equatorial Guinea International Prize for research in Life Sciences at Paris. He has also received the Dr Lee Jong-Wook Memorial Prize for Public Health, 2019 by the WHO, Geneva. Last year, he received the President's Gold Medal from the Royal College of Physicians, Glasgow. He has been awarded the 'Padma Shri' high civilian award by the Honourable President of India.

GOING VIRAL

MAKING OF COVAXIN:
THE INSIDE STORY

BALRAM BHARGAVA

RUPA

Published by
Rupa Publications India Pvt. Ltd 2021
7/16, Ansari Road, Daryaganj
New Delhi 110002

Sales centres:
Allahabad Bengaluru Chennai
Hyderabad Jaipur Kathmandu
Kolkata Mumbai

Copyright © Balram Bhargava 2021

ISBN: 978-93-5520-022-8

Third impression 2022

10 9 8 7 6 5 4 3

The moral right of the author has been asserted.

Printed at Thomson Press India Ltd, Faridabad

Dedicated to
Health professionals, essential services workers, security
forces, nameless civil servants burning the midnight oil and
countless people from all walks of life who have contributed
to bravely fighting the grave battle against this
once-in-a-century pandemic.

CONTENTS

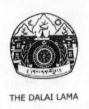

THE DALAI LAMA

FOREWORD

The COVID-19 pandemic has caused much misery throughout the world. However, it is crucial that we not lose hope. When faced with difficulties, it is particularly important to garner courage and determination. Consistent effort is, I believe, the proper way to deal with challenges.

Around the world, scientists, doctors, nurses and many other front-line workers have been risking their own lives to help save the lives of others. I truly appreciate their heroic and selfless efforts.

As we are all so interconnected and dependent on one another, the well-being of others is our concern. We must maintain sight of the oneness of humanity. Our genuine sense of concern for others—our altruistic attitude—is the source of our own happiness, as compassion develops our inner strength, which brings about our inner peace.

The hard work of scientists has led to the development of vaccines within a very short time. The success of our Indian scientists in developing this country's own vaccine is commendable. The successes at various levels are due to the immense capabilities of our scientists, health professionals and the many others involved, and reflect strong, clear leadership.

Going Viral records the encouraging story of tackling the pandemic in India and the efforts of all who have worked tirelessly to keep us safe. I hope this book will help us appreciate their achievements.

14 September 2021

His Holiness the 14th Dalai Lama

Prologue
TAKING THE BULL BY THE HORNS

On 30 January 2020, India detected its first case of COVID-19 in a student in Kerala.[1] We hit the ground running thereafter. In less than two months, by 20 March, it became the fifth country in the world to successfully isolate the SARS-CoV-2 virus strain. On 18 May, India reached a landmark in its fight against COVID-19 by performing 100,000 COVID-19 tests in a single day.[2] And on 16 January 2021, the country began its roll out of Covaxin, a home-grown vaccine.[3] Less than a year after a completely unknown disease appeared, we had the means to tame its severity.

In this book, I attempt to tell a story, albeit a true one, with twists and turns that can make for a good thriller. And much like a Bollywood film, this story too has moments of exhilaration and tragedy.

In December 2019, when the world woke up to the ominous news of an emerging pandemic, nobody knew exactly how it would play out.[4] But the forecasts were dire. None of us had ever faced anything like it. None of us felt prepared, but we had to step up. Naturally, we were apprehensive in India, given the less than satisfactory state of our health infrastructure.

But we began work immediately, getting all the elements for a robust response in place—from the science needed, to the logistics of dealing with a disaster of this magnitude. Figuring out the genomic map of the new virus,[5] creating the reagents (substances that help detect a virus) to produce testing kits, setting up a national network of diagnostic laboratories,[6][7] examining potential therapeutics and, most importantly, developing an effective vaccine. In December 2019, I was a cardiologist above all else. Now, I can claim to having studied in the hard, real school of public health and crisis management. The experience turned me into an author too.

While the progress in science, along with the early nationwide lockdown, helped reduce the impact of the pandemic considerably, we suffered greatly as a nation. By early 2021, after a slow start, India had recorded the third-largest number of cases and also the third-highest COVID-19 death toll in the world.[8]

However, the figures per million of those infected or of mortality due to COVID-19, were relatively low compared to many higher income countries.[9] For example, on 3 January 2021, India's deaths per million was 109, compared to 903 in the United States (US), 1,036 in Italy and 1,524 in Belgium.[10]

Unfortunately, in April 2021, the situation took a turn for the worse for India and many other countries that had escaped the first wave of COVID-19 relatively unscathed.

During the second wave, we were much better informed but not necessarily better prepared. The new variant with the rapid spread of the disease and a higher oxygen demand in the patients overwhelmed the infrastructure. Too many people suffered or died. Even a single death is one too many.

In this book, I have tried to describe, in as easy a language as possible, the phenomenal work that our scientists, administrators, healthcare workers, various central and state agencies and private sector collaborators did to keep India safe. It is an attempt to relate some of the long-term investments, work and people who made it possible for us to navigate our way to the ultimate goal—a vaccine to put an end to the horror.

I readily admit that there have been shortcomings and mistakes. However, it is also important to document our successes. As the director general of the Indian Council of Medical Research (ICMR) and author, this book is my tribute to every single person who has worked, and continues to work, round the clock, putting themselves and their families at risk for no other reward than to serve their country. It is my ode to my incredible colleagues and their counterparts in scientific institutions elsewhere, who helped create the COVID-19 vaccine we are using now, along with a variety of other technologies critical to controlling and rolling back the pandemic.

I am not a public health specialist, but we have an

excellent team of public health specialists at the ICMR that guided me. Decision-making, particularly on major issues, was tough at times. It is difficult to take everyone along even in times of crisis.

The other major strength of the ICMR, which I have observed being an outsider who joined only three years ago, is that this organization has a tremendous history and tradition, being one of the oldest research bodies in the world. It is the country's apex body for the formulation, coordination and promotion of research in medicine and biology. Its 27 national institutes are engaged in research on diseases, both contagious and otherwise. This includes tuberculosis, cholera, malaria, water-borne diseases and AIDS. The ICMR is also involved in issues of nutrition, occupational health, reproductive health, tribal health, medical statistics, implementation research, etc. Its research priorities are in tandem with the country's health policies as laid down from time to time by the government.

Thus, the ICMR regularly deals with outbreak investigations and is ready to meet any challenge, however formidable. I was able to leverage this capacity during the pandemic and had the occasion to admire the resilience of my team members.

On a personal note, I am compelled to note that after being part of every aspect, from transportation logistics to bat research, it is hard to describe how privileged I feel. Yes, it has been an incredibly stressful time of heavy responsibility, constant pivoting and of choosing work over sleep and family. But—and I'm sure my fellow team members share this feeling—I have never felt more useful, or more engaged.

Let me clarify that this book is not a thorough analysis of every aspect of India's responses to the Covid pandemic. That is yet to be done and will be done, at some point, in great technical detail to help us understand our strengths and weaknesses and prepare better for the future.

For the time being, it is important for everyone, especially the citizens of this great nation, to understand all that has been achieved already by our institutions and the sacrifices people working on the front lines of the pandemic have made to keep them safe from the pandemic.

As I write these words, the virus still lurks. Reports of its new variants are most worrisome. We cannot let our guard down. But even while I see a nation and a world in agony, I have witnessed instances of courage and brilliance. The young people who risked their lives to fly and rescue their fellow Indians; the scientists who handled a virus that could easily have killed them; the innovators who figured out how to make all the moving parts fit so that we could organize testing, tracking and treating. Honoured and humbled, I have a duty to narrate some of those incredible stories.

As the pandemic continues to hold us in its vicious grip, the remarkable story of the development of Covaxin could serve as a model for how to prepare for future challenges. There will be many until we get our act together and preserve mother Earth—protect our forests and prevent global warming!

1

PREPARING FOR THE APOCALYPSE

t all began in December 2019, when Chinese officials notified the World Health Organization (WHO) about a terrifying new virus. Health authorities around the globe sat up and took notice.[1]

In India, the Ministry of Health and Family Welfare (MoHFW), the ICMR and other government agencies followed the unfolding situation in China through the WHO's regular bulletins. We were concerned, but not unduly alarmed. After all, India had hardly been impacted by the severe acute respiratory syndrome (SARS) outbreak a decade and half ago, and in more recent years, very successfully tackled both the Zika and Nipah virus outbreaks. We believed that we could effectively tackle the new virus, if it came to that.

In early January 2020, India put in place policy measures, personnel and systems needed to respond to the threat posed by the novel coronavirus—SARS-CoV-2, which causes a disease named COVID-19. The MoHFW set up a round-the-clock control room to continuously assess the preparedness and response mechanisms to manage any case that might get imported to India. A control room was set up at the ICMR headquarters to ramp up testing and keep tabs on new research evidence across the globe.

People infected with COVID-19 typically remain infectious for up to 10 days in moderate cases and two weeks in severe cases. We developed and disseminated a surveillance plan for tackling COVID-19 on 25 January, five days before the WHO declared it an international public health emergency. We identified hospitals with isolation facilities near all international airports and kept them in a state of preparedness to meet any emergency requirements, with necessary stocks of protective gear and trained personnel.

State governments across the country were also requested to review their preparedness to deal with the pandemic. They were asked to identify gaps and strengthen core capacities in surveillance, lab support, infection prevention and control, and to pay special attention to hospital preparedness in terms of isolation and ventilator management of critically ill patients.

We had already initiated thermal screening in mid-January for all airline passengers coming from China, Hong Kong, Singapore and Thailand, at 21 international airports around the country. Subsequently, India launched graded restrictions on international travel from affected countries, moving on to quarantine strategies at ports of entry, testing for COVID-19 and implementing social distancing measures. The WHO officially declared COVID-19 a pandemic and a public health emergency of international concern on 11 March 2020, well after we had taken several preventive measures.

THE FIRST CASE

The first case of COVID-19 infection came from Kerala on 30 January. That first patient was one of a batch of students who had returned home from Wuhan, China, where they had been studying medicine. With panic setting in slowly all around, it was a long and tortuous journey for them as they went from Wuhan to Kolkata and finally Kochi, where they were detected with COVID-19 by the ICMR's National Institute of Virology (NIV) while in isolation.

Dr Priya Abraham, director, NIV recalls:

On the night of 29 January, I was on my way to Pune after a meeting in Delhi. I was at the airport terminal when one of our scientists called me and said, 'Ma'am. I think we have a positive.' I said, 'Okay, has the other lab taken it up?' I had lined up two labs for COVID-19 testing. One was the primary lab, and the other was to verify the findings of the first in a blinded manner, so that we could be doubly sure of the results we generated. I arrived in Pune at 10.30 p.m. and headed straight to the Institute. I went through all the data—by then the second lab had also come up with their results. As per the results generated by both laboratories, we had a positive.

It was a dramatic night with very little margin for error, and I am thankful to the team for its promptness and the hard work its members put in. We cross-checked the data repeatedly, working late into the night, discussing and reviewing the data. The gravity of the results of our testing was huge—to tell the government, the people of the country and the world, that the virus had entered our shores. Dr Raman Gangakhedkar, a senior scientist from the ICMR was then on a visit to the institute, and we reported the matter to him. He in turn reported it to the government, and the rest is history.

The immediate reaction at that point in time on 30 January, our martyrdom day, was a sort of worry as well. When you give someone bad news, then you are kind of going in to a shell for some time. It just took time for us to absorb it.

At that point, though we were not very clear about the seriousness of the disease, we knew that it was a problem. It was something that had the potential to develop in a big way, big enough for the world to be alarmed. It could be something like SARS or Middle East respiratory syndrome (MERS), and there could be a first wave, then a second... even a third. The pandemic had begun to bare its fangs in most of Europe and the US. Europe had already begun to report large mortalities. We then knew that we had a crisis on our hands—one that we had not encountered in almost a century.

For India especially, the problem was even graver. We do not have the best of health infrastructure. As a nation with 1.3 billion people, we have faced several challenges upgrading our health system over the decades. Increasing population, leading to a severely burdened public health sector, thus rising dependence on the private system, was one of them. The public healthcare system had been a great relief to the financially needy since the government, through the taxpayers' money, had taken care of their requirements. The private sector, on the other hand, charged amounts that were non-affordable to the vast majority of the population.

While the private system catered to those who could afford the costs, the aim of universal health coverage could not be met through private involvement alone, although they are a critical component in the country's overall health infrastructure. We needed to get our act together and put in place restrictive measures. We had to take advantage of what we had at hand and therefore, using our resources judiciously, we were able to manage the first wave. We took cues from the Western countries and effectively model our responses with our frugal mindset. At the start of the pandemic, no one had any idea about how to manage the disease. If you look closely at the number of cases and deaths in most Western and well-developed countries, even with state-of-the-art health infrastructure, they had a very high death rate. So, we had to take the toughest decision to implement a massive nationwide lockdown at that point in time and use that timeframe to ramp up our health resources effectively.

GETTING STARTED

The Government of India swung into action once the gravity of the new pandemic began to sink in. There were issues relating to quarantining people from outside the country. There were several pressing questions that needed to be settled. How many travellers would be tested and quarantined? How and where would the quarantine centres come up? How would our Armed Forces and paramilitary forces be involved and how would they create quarantine centres? A series of meetings were regularly held for the creation of quarantine centres, and the government moved at a rapid speed. Data collected over the days was presented to the GoM.

We, at the ICMR, had our first interaction with top leadership and higher officials when proposed in the first week of March that all international flights be stopped and every single traveller be tested.

We made a presentation of eight to 10 slides which highlighted the roadmap to tackle the crisis.

We were asked to give our recommendations on a white paper. And we wrote two lines on that paper:

1. Impose a lockdown
2. Stop all international travel

As Indian health officials, we knew this much: the virus would inevitably wreak havoc. It was highly contagious, and because many of those infected were asymptomatic, it was near impossible to control.

A national task force for COVID-19 was constituted within the ICMR. We got in touch with the foremost names in epidemiology and virology, in operations research and in pharmacology and public health in India, and made them part of the task force.

Since the task force's inception, we've had nearly 150 meetings. The various subgroups dealt with policy decisions, as well as decisions related to sero-survey, case management, diagnostic algorithm and how to tackle socio-behavioural issues.

The Government of India showed tremendous faith in us right from the beginning. It went along with our suggestions, which we gave from time to time. They trusted us on the science and the data that we presented.

Further, the ICMR had a strong track record of dealing with outbreaks and epidemics like H1N1, Nipah, Zika and others. Even the biosafety level 4 (BSL-4) laboratory, the highest containment system to deal with the deadliest of viruses, was created in the ICMR system for the first time in Asia, at the National Institute of Virology (NIV), Pune, in 2012, followed by the Wuhan Lab in 2017.

In preparation of the approaching storm, the Union government imposed a nationwide lockdown starting from 24 March. It was the most effective of its kind anywhere in the world; a balanced one, compared to the very stringent one in China and a very lax one in the West—Buddha's middle path. This gave our health authorities valuable time to prepare for the worst that was yet to come.

As we were the main agency, initially guiding the nation during the pandemic, I had a sense of responsibility as well as fear, as I had never dealt with such a major catastrophe. I had to anticipate and act swiftly, and my training as a physician as well as a cardiologist helped me immensely. More than 30 years in a public sector hospital have kept me in touch with the reality and suffering of a large number of our people.

I have been fortunate enough to treat nearly a quarter million patients during my life. During my career as a physician, being able to bring a smile on the face of patients or their relatives had always helped me cope with the challenges. This new experience was a much larger problem with no immediate smiles. However, the satisfaction of innovating, improvising, repurposing and calibrating the responses with results did boost my morale.

LOCKDOWN CONSTRAINTS

When we were in lockdown, our mantra was to keep the windows open and the doors shut. All the knowledge would come in and we would consolidate that knowledge from different parts of the world and make a decision. During the lockdown, one of our major concerns for uninterrupted response planning was our colleagues' safety. The ICMR guest house in New Delhi was being used as a bubble zone, taking care of scientists and technicians while they worked till 2.00 a.m. arranging for shipments of diagnostic kits to different parts of the country. Fortunately, we were able to get insurance for all our lab staff.

For me, life at home was the biggest stress buster. Both my sons are also physicians and were involved in Covid care. They often came up with suggestions and novel ideas that the ICMR could adopt to keep India safe. It was a great help. My wife and daughter-in-law were all at home during the lockdown and would run the kitchen with joy and innovation and worked from home. Every evening there would be a family meal, when we shared all our daily news and experiences with grace and a thank you to the Almighty. It was a bonus for me to have everyone together during the lockdown, it helped keep me sane. Of course, my family was worried that I was interacting with so many people all day, thus increasing the risk for myself. But it was my duty which I could not shirk from. Before

Covid, I never slept with my cellphone by my bedside and never used WhatsApp, but that has changed now. I had to be connected round the clock. Generally I slept well, but many times I would get some ideas in the middle of the night or early in the morning, which I would note down on a pad.

Depending on the situation and gravity at that particular frame of time, my day would go on till 8 or 9 p.m., even after 10 at times. We were always trying to find mechanisms by which India could demonstrate its leadership in this period of crisis.

The ICMR has published around 250 research papers, several guidelines and advisories during the last one and a half years, just on COVID. It indicates the kind of effort that went on in the ICMR across India, in different ICMR laboratories and institutions.

A similar situation existed for our scientists at all our institutes, particularly the NIV, Pune, where they were conducting experiments at all hours, every day. Staff from various other institutes was involved in collecting samples for the sero-surveys while the rapid analysis was done at the National Institute of Epidemiology (NIE), guiding the pandemic response. The entire ICMR staff did not let me down even for a minute. They put in unearthly hours.

Faced with an unprecedented challenge, both in terms of technicality and scale, Indian scientists had to innovate extensively, health workers had to train and learn on the job, administrators had to coordinate amid the challenges of a nationwide lockdown and civil and defence aviation personnel had to fly at the shortest of notices.

Then the inevitable happened: the few cases of COVID-19 grew to a few hundred and then to a few thousand until the trickle became a flood, growing rapidly after May 2020, and reaching a peak of nearly 1 lakh cases every day in September 2020, before beginning to slowly decline.

As part of the first wave of the pandemic, India had recorded the third-largest number of cases and also the third-highest COVID-19 death toll in the world in absolute numbers, although the case fatality rate in the country was remarkably low compared to many higher income nations.[2][3][4] By mid-March 2021, India had recorded a total of 11.5 million cases, while the death toll stood at over 159,000. By this time, COVID-19 had also spread phenomenally around the globe, infecting over 109 million people, resulting in more than 2.4 million deaths since the start of the pandemic.

This changed for the worse during our second wave, which started sometime in February 2021, reaching its peak in May 2021, and then gradually started declining in most of the states. By 12 June 2021, India had the second-largest number of cases in the world at 29.4 million and total deaths had more than doubled, within just a couple of months, to 370,168. On the same day, the total number of cases worldwide stood at nearly 176.4 million, with 3.8 million deaths.

However, horrifying as these morbidity and mortality numbers are, they don't even begin to tell the story of the pain that the global and Indian population has borne. Hundreds of thousands lives lost, children orphaned, families separated, jobs gone, education decimated, health destroyed, symptoms so terrible that you cannot bear them alone and yet you must, as you are dying alone with no loved ones allowed near you. We are just beginning to find out about the long-term damage to our hearts, lungs, brains, psyches, economies and the future.

The pandemic has served to highlight and identify the gaps in our healthcare system. This is the time, more than ever, to evaluate our system and responses. We must prepare for the future. The government has, over the years, launched several healthcare initiatives, such as the National Health Mission, Ayushman Bharat Yojana, Mission Indradhanush and the Integrated Child Development Services. These have all served to ramp up our healthcare infrastructure, but much more needs to be done and is being done on war footing.

A good way to begin reforms is to allot more investments in healthcare, both preventive and in the area of treatment. While it is true that expenditure on public health has seen a rise in the recent years, it is still woefully short of the target of 2.5 per cent of the country's GDP.

An increase in investments in healthcare is not enough though. It must be accompanied by speeding up key policy efforts around public sector reforms, mainly in the area of infrastructure.

COVID-19 was the first pandemic of this century to hit the country, but it will not be the last. We must prepare for the future now and the government is committed and is monitoring the rapid development.

2

CORONAVIRUS:
THE SCIENCE EXPLAINED

W hat is a virus? And how has it become a source of such death and destruction?

A virus is made up of a core of genetic material, either ribonucleic acid (RNA) or of deoxyribonucleic acid (DNA). It is surrounded by a protective coat called a capsid, made up of protein. SARS-CoV-2 is an RNA virus. RNA viruses are generally more volatile and mutate faster than DNA viruses.

Is a virus a living thing? Maybe. Sometimes. It depends on its location. A viral particle is inert unless it is in a host cell. On its own, it cannot reproduce itself or do much of anything at all. Once it makes itself comfortable in a host cell, it can bring the world to its knees, as we are witnessing.

Viruses are the most abundant biological entities on planet Earth. The best current estimate is that there are a whopping 10^{30} virus particles in the biosphere. If all the viruses on Earth were laid end to end, they would stretch for 100 million light years.[1] Unbelievable but true!

The virus responsible for COVID-19 is suspected to be of zoonotic origin—transmitted between animals and people. An estimated 60 per cent of known infectious diseases and 75 per cent of all new, emerging or re-emerging diseases in humans have origins in animals.[2] However, other theories about the origin of the coronavirus are still under investigation.

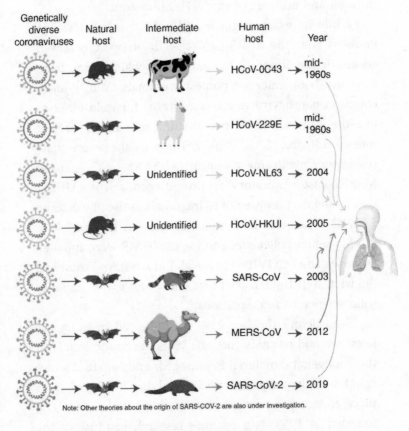

Note: Other theories about the origin of SARS-COV-2 are also under investigation.

Figure 2.1: Coronaviruses that affect humans

Apart from COVID-19 and the Nipah virus disease (NVD), a variety of other zoonotic diseases, including avian influenza, Crimean-Congo haemorrhagic fever (CCHF) and Zika, have recently emerged as threats to public health in India and are part of the WHO blueprint.[3]

While its exact origin is still unknown, what we do know is that the SARS-CoV-2 is the newest of seven coronaviruses found in humans, all of which came from animals—bats, mice or domestic animals. While many common coronaviruses are responsible for mild illnesses like the common cold, two in the same family are far more deadly than SARS-CoV-2. These are the severe acute respiratory syndrome coronavirus (SARS-CoV) and the Middle East respiratory syndrome coronavirus (MERS-CoV). Luckily, they are not as infectious as the one causing COVID-19, so the death toll they cause is limited.

My senior colleagues and I at the ICMR were appalled as we watched COVID-19 spread. But we stayed calm and did what well-trained scientists know best to do—dip into solid science to find solutions.

Even before the first case was detected in India, we knew we had to study the new virus's genomic sequence (how its genetic material is arranged) and isolate it so we could start figuring out ways to subdue it. The obvious place to do this exercise was the NIV Pune. The NIV, founded in 1953, is a premier research institute of the ICMR and a WHO Collaborating Centre.

As ICMR's premier testing facility, for a variety of viral diseases and with a staff that had successfully dealt with several infectious disease outbreaks in the past, the entire country was depending on NIV to deliver. Until this premier BSL-4 facility was set up in 2012, all samples of virus testing were sent to the US. Apart from the hard science required to isolate the virus, culture it in the lab, understand its characteristics—which was critical later for vaccine development—NIV scientists also played a vital role in helping ramp up testing throughout the country, under tremendous pressure.

Just two years before COVID-19, an outbreak of the deadly Nipah virus in Kerala in 2018, provided valuable experience to NIV scientists in handling high-risk viruses, developing rapid diagnostic kits and framing various protocols for containing the spread of infectious disease in communities.

The NVD was one of the WHO's top eight emerging pathogens in 2017.[4] The virus struck the Kozhikode and Malappuram districts, claiming 21 lives out of a total 23 cases—a case fatality rate (CFR) of close to 90 per cent.[5] As of now, we have no vaccines or approved therapy for NVD, which has an average incubation period in humans of 4–14 days.[6]

During the 2018 outbreak, the NIV managed to isolate the Nipah virus at its high-security facilities. In 2019, scientists there developed the first-ever indigenous point-of-care (PoC) test for the virus, using serological and nucleic acid amplification techniques.

This dramatically reduced the time taken to test human samples for the Nipah virus to just under an hour. In the absence of such a PoC testing device, samples had to be physically transported to the NIV lab in Pune for testing, taking a minimum of 24 hours to get the results. The delay naturally caused much anxiety to patients as well as the health authorities. Later, the PoC test kits were also deployed in neighbouring Bangladesh as part of the research studies on Nipah outbreaks.

NIV scientists retrieved the complete genome of SARS-CoV-2 from the students who had returned from Wuhan, and among whom was India's first Covid positive case. Scientists found that it accurately matched that of the virus found among patients in Wuhan. Decoding the virus was the first, small but vital, step in understanding its structure and understanding both its strengths and weaknesses. The information was also crucial in developing new diagnostics, designing new medicines to treat COVID-19 patients, following the mutations of the virus as they occurred and, most importantly, developing a vaccine.

'We understood that once we had the virus in hand, then it will open an arena of opportunities in terms of developing diagnostics, testing monoclonal antibodies and doing several other animal challenge experiments for therapeutics and vaccines,' Dr Nivedita Gupta, my colleague who heads the virology unit of the ICMR, remarked.

But this was easier said than done. Apart from shortages of essential materials needed to develop tests or conduct analyses, in the first couple of months of 2020, there was also a lack of sufficient samples from COVID-19 patients to work with.

'The first few months of the pandemic were the most frustrating ones, as we felt completely helpless against the new virus,' remembers Dr Pragya Yadav, lead researcher and in-charge of the BSL-4 lab at NIV Pune, which handles the most pathogenic viruses.

ISOLATING THE VIRUS

Isolating the virus was an even more technically demanding procedure. To start with, we required high-quality samples from people infected with SARS-CoV-2. To be of any use, the samples had to have a high viral load, and someone had to get them safely to NIV's laboratory. All of this finally happened in the middle of March, when 12 samples—eight from Italian tourists[7] and their contacts in New Delhi and four from Agra[8]—became available.

'The samples arrived at our lab only past midnight, around 2.00 a.m. Our team was waiting and immediately got to work,' recalls Dr Yadav, highlighting the sense of urgency that her team of scientists felt at that time to get on with cracking the mystery of the new virus.

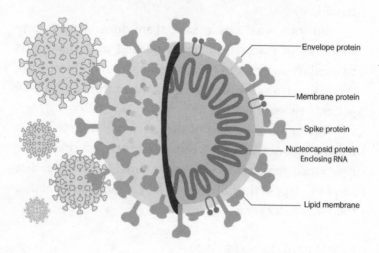

Figure 2.2: The SARS-CoV-2 structure

The scientists used the samples to try and grow the SARS-CoV-2 virus in the lab. If you think this sounds tricky, you're right. The NIV team managed it by infusing the samples into Vero cells, which are harvested from the kidneys of African green monkeys and make a good medium for growing all kinds of viruses.

Once the virus attaches itself to the Vero cell, it starts multiplying inside and then begins to spread from one cell to another at an exponential rate. The growing load of the virus changes the shape of the cells and often even kills them, a phenomenon that seen under a microscope, looks like a bizarre piece of science fiction becoming a reality.

However, to confirm that the virus involved is really SARS-CoV-2 and not any other, technicians must carry out a round of genomic sequencing of the 'virus soup' produced. Then they can compare the genetic structure of the lab-cultured virus with information from other studies.

When the NIV researchers isolated the virus,[9] they could produce large quantities of the organism whenever needed. All this took place within one week, with scientists working round the clock. On the final day, the team was at it until 5.00 a.m.

'It was quite a challenge, but we were successful in getting around 11 strains of the virus isolated. Now, we could start some real research,' Dr Yadav said. India was the fifth country to successfully isolate the virus strain after China, Japan, Thailand and the US.

THE BADA SAAB OF THE PANDEMIC

If there were ever a competition for deceptive looks, SARS-CoV-2 would win hands down. 'It's a pretty virus!' exclaimed Dr Priya Abraham, director, NIV, whose researchers at the institute were the first team in India to identify the virus under an electron microscope[10] and decipher its genomic structure. The 'prettiness' comes from the spike-like structures that sit on top of the virus and look like a 'corona' or crown, a common characteristic of the entire family of coronaviruses to which it belongs.

As mentioned earlier, viruses, unlike other microbes such as bacteria or fungal pathogens, cannot survive on their own without a host cell to infect. Viruses must get inside cells of other living organisms and use the biochemical machinery of those cells to build new virus particles, replicate and spread themselves.

Human cells have their own protective mechanisms to ward off such invasions by viruses, such as a fatty layer that holds in all the enzymes, proteins and DNA that make up a cell. Viruses such as SARS-CoV-2 must get past this barrier to enter the human cell. They do this by using proteins or glycoproteins on their surface to fuse their own membrane to that of the host cell and take it over.

The protein that SARS-CoV-2 uses to get into human cells is shaped like a spike, which sticks out from the surface of the envelope around the virus. These spikes attach themselves to a protein on the surface of human cells called angiotensin-converting enzyme 2 or ACE2, commonly found in our lungs, heart, intestines, blood vessels and muscles.[11]

While the spike proteins help the virus attach to human cells and gain entry to propagate itself, they are also its weakest spots. Many antiviral vaccines target the spike protein on the SARS-CoV-2 virus by helping the human immune system produce protective antibodies.

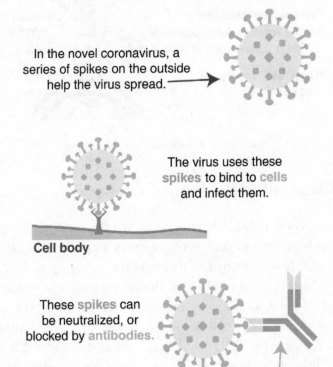

Figure 2.3: How SARS-CoV-2 gets into cells and reproduces[12]

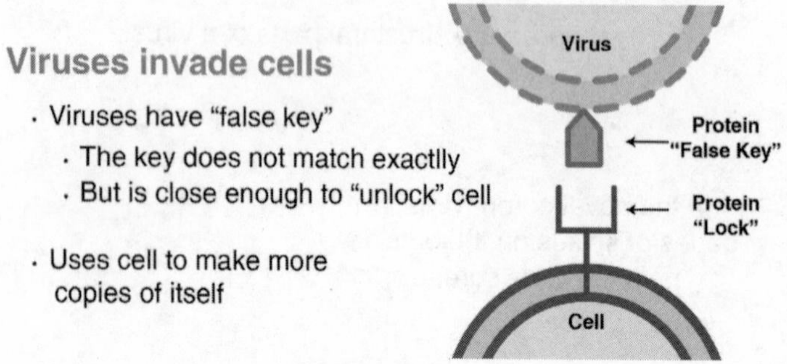
Viruses invade cells
Viruses have "false key"
The key does not match exactlly
But is close enough to "unlock" cell
Uses cell to make more copies of itself
Virus
Protein "False Key"
Protein "Lock"
Cell

Figure 2.4: The 'Lock and Key' mechanism

INSIDE NIV'S HIGH-SECURITY LAB

The NIV's BSL-4 laboratory can handle most kinds of highly infectious and exotic viruses impacting human health. It was the first of its kind in Asia, set up in 2012.

Setting up the BSL-4 lab almost a decade ago was an act of great foresight by the leadership of the ICMR at that time. China's first BSL-4 lab in Wuhan, the epicentre of the global COVID-19 outbreak, came up only in 2017.

Biosafety levels (BSL) are used to identify the protective measures needed in a laboratory setting, to protect workers, the environment and the public. Activities and projects conducted in biological laboratories are categorized for their biosafety levels. The four levels are BSL-1, BSL-2, BSL-3 and BSL-4, with BSL-4 being the highest (maximum) level of containment.

While dealing with biological hazards at this level, the use of protective gear and a self-contained oxygen supply is mandatory. The entrance and exit of a level four bio-laboratory contain multiple showers, a vacuum room and other safety precautions designed to destroy all traces of the biohazard.

'Not every ordinary lab can do this,' Dr Abraham observed. 'It's very high security.'

Multiple airlocks are employed and electronically secured to prevent both doors opening at the same time. All air and water service going to and coming from a BSL-4 lab must undergo similar decontamination procedures to eliminate the possibility of an accidental release of microorganisms. Access to BSL-4 laboratories is carefully controlled and requires significant training. No virus can be allowed to go out into the environment, even during the most adverse conditions like an earthquake.

Such intimidating scenes that we see in scary films about killer viruses are part of daily life in a BSL-4 lab.

One of the immediate benefits of isolating and producing the SARS-CoV-2 virus in large quantities in the lab was that it helped in the development of diagnostic kits to detect antibodies produced by the human body against the infection. In the early phase of the pandemic, India was dependent on import of the antibody testing kits, mostly from China.

In April 2020, we decided to conduct the first

sero-prevalance survey to understand the extent of the spread in India. This required mass production of antibody testing kits, which look for antibodies in a blood sample to determine if an individual has had a past infection with the virus that causes COVID-19. Antibody tests were a rare feat in April 2020, not just in India but also globally. It was a challenging process. I gave the responsibility of developing these testing kits to my colleagues at NIV Pune. Since we were running short on time, antibody testing kits had to be developed within a week's time without compromising on quality. This seemed like an impossible task, but the team did it!

The BSL-4 team grew the virus and standardized the Enzyme-Linked Immunosorbent Assay (ELISA).[13] The assay is a plate-based technique to detect and quantify soluble substances such as peptides, proteins, antibodies and hormones. The NIV team[14] made a panel for validation of this assay, and finally our scientists successfully developed India's first indigenous kit for COVID-19 antibody detection, which used the ELISA method. This was a huge achievement, as we were able to launch our own testing kits when similar kits imported from abroad were failing and providing unreliable results.

The antibody tests, unlike the reverse transcription polymerase chain reaction (RT-PCR) test that is done on nasal/throat swabs or in saliva, are carried out on blood samples. Also, while the RT-PCR tests are carried out only on patients who might be currently infected, with or without symptoms, antibody tests detect whether one was infected with SARS-COV-2 in the past. This is because those who get infected carry antibodies produced by their immune systems for several months, if not years, after recovery. So, while RT-PCR tests show up as negative once the acute viral infection is over, the antibody tests can still show positive results even among individuals who did not develop symptoms during acute attack.

The NIV transferred the know-how to Indian companies for manufacture. The ICMR signed MoUs with seven Indian companies for the transfer of technology and mass production of the kits. The first kit, 'CovidKavach ELISA', was launched in May 2020, by the Ahmedabad-based Zydus Cadila, which worked closely with the NIV team to ensure high quality.

The development and scaled-up production of the CovidKavach ELISA kits was a genuine team effort between government bodies, the private sector and a variety of research institutions. The ICMR headquarters helped speed up clearances, and Zydus Cadila and other private manufacturers did the commercialization.

Since the country was under a complete lockdown, it was challenging for Cadila to procure the key components for the development of the kit, such as sealers and lyophilizers, which are generally imported. 'We were in a fix,' recalled Dr Gupta. 'The industry does not work on borrowing material for producing kits from different suppliers, but we were operating during a public health emergency. I remember reaching out to the Serum Institute of India to arrange sealers. NIV gave lyophilizers and this is how the first batch of antibody testing kits came about in India! We also successfully met the deadline that our leadership had given us.'

The kits were put to immediate use by the ICMR's National Institute of Epidemiology in Chennai, which led several rounds of country-wide sero-surveys along with 15 other ICMR institutes. These surveys, done at four different phases of the pandemic in both urban and rural settings,[15] were the largest of their kind anywhere in the world, and helped the Indian government and health authorities adjust strategy according to what we found.

The sero-survey data, by detecting people with antibodies of COVID-19, gave us a reasonably good idea of what percentage of the population may have developed immunity.[16] [17] [18] In the long run and in the absence of a vaccine, more and more people acquiring antibodies was the only way the pandemic would slow down.

We, at the ICMR, never thought that the idea of 'herd immunity' through infections was a good one, contrary to what some experts in other countries and even in India seemed to suggest. We knew that protecting the elderly and people with comorbidities, in a densely populated country like ours, while only the young got infected, was next to impossible.

We all know that every Indian professes to be a physician. My worst moments were when I was approached with all kinds of remedies and cures without biological plausibility to be tested for antiviral properties with the limited resources at NIV.

The priority from April 2020 onwards was to quickly develop the vaccine and not search for unproven therapies in the dark.

3
TESTING TIMES

How do you control an infection? Detect. Isolate. Treat. Trace contacts. Manage. Prevent.

In the absence of an effective treatment, prevention is the best strategy, and it revolves around testing. That's where the challenge lay. How do we cover 1.3 billion people, and that too in a short time, since the pandemic was spreading rapidly? But inclusive and equitable access to testing was essential. So, we had to optimize our limited resources based on the evolving epidemic so that we could scale up sustainably.

In early February 2020, as the pandemic slowly began to gain a foothold in India, only one laboratory in the country was testing for COVID-19—one at NIV Pune. In this story of superheroes, the NIV, part of our ICMR family, is the first one. Worryingly, all testing kits and reagents were being imported from outside the country. We had to do something dramatic to change the situation and we did.

Over a period of five months, the number of laboratories in the country performing RT-PCR tests for diagnosing COVID-19 rose to more than 1,596 in August 2020.[1] More than half a dozen Indian manufacturers were making the RT-PCR test kits.

On 18 May, India reached a landmark in its fight against COVID-19 by performing 100,000 COVID-19 tests in a single day. Starting from less than 100 tests per day only two months earlier, this represented a thousand-fold increase in just 60 days. It was a historic achievement in the annals of India's public health. By January 2021, a whopping 1.4 million people were being tested every day. The world sat up and took notice.

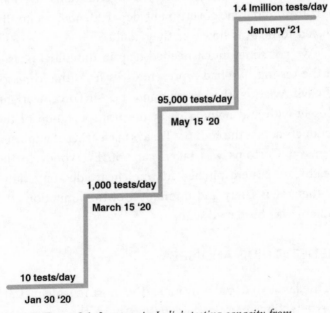

Figure 3.1. Increase in India's testing capacity from January 2020 to January 2021

'India's testing capabilities now match that of the advanced countries,' Dr Roderico H. Ofrin, the WHO's representative to India, remarked.

The remarkable story of how India became fully self-reliant in its testing capabilities in such a short time begins and ends with the sheer commitment of dedicated teams from research institutions, medical colleges, testing laboratories, ministries, airlines and postal services working together. The Government of India helped us immensely in coordinating amongst different organizations. We had staff from different government departments specifically posted to help us however they could.

We got some much-needed help in the initial phases of the testing. We had representatives from the Ministry of Civil Aviation, the railways and the Air Force, working closely with and helping us in the transportation of the products across the country. Delays in clearing of imported items at Customs was taken care of. Everybody in the healthcare system pitched in wholeheartedly, unmindful of their own safety and unmindful of the limitations the system was burdened with.

GENETIC HIDE-AND-SEEK

In the last two decades or more, the most reliable method for detecting many pathogens has been the polymerase chain reaction or PCR, a process that very rapidly makes multiple copies of a specific DNA sample. This allows scientists to amplify very small samples of DNA and study them in detail to understand their origins and characteristics.

However, some viruses such as the SARS-CoV-2 contain only RNA and no DNA. To detect such a virus, scientists need to convert the RNA to DNA through a process called 'reverse transcription'—which is what the RT in the RT-PCR tests, widely used to detect COVID-19, stands for. The RT-PCR method involves the use of several reagents, called primers, probes and positive controls, that help identify the presence or absence of a specific virus.

In the initial stages of the pandemic, given the paucity of both testing equipment and trained personnel, and our high dependence on imported materials, we decided to follow a highly calibrated testing strategy devised by the country's National Task Force (NTF) for COVID-19.

Starting in late January 2020, with the screening of air passengers arriving from countries most affected by COVID-19,[2] testing was expanded in phases to include contacts of infected travellers, healthcare workers and all cases of severe respiratory or influenza-like illness in the country.

As domestic capacity expanded with the induction of new testing platforms, the Indian health system went from catering to only prioritized sections of the population to making testing available on demand for everyone.

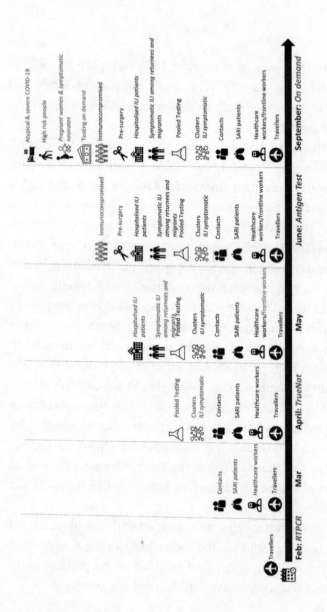

Figure 3.2: Calibrated expansion of testing

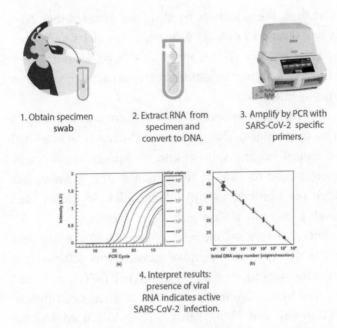

1. Obtain specimen swab

2. Extract RNA from specimen and convert to DNA.

3. Amplify by PCR with SARS-CoV-2 specific primers.

4. Interpret results: presence of viral RNA indicates active SARS-CoV-2 infection.

Figure 3.3: RT-PCR or molecular tests for detecting COVID-19

A team of scientists at NIV Pune, had begun preparing to put together all the reagents needed to detect the SARS-CoV-2 virus as soon as news about the outbreak was broadcast worldwide in late December 2019. We did not know when the disease would finally arrive on Indian territory. But, knowing how pandemics have worked in the past, we knew it was only a matter of time. Readiness was an imperative, not a choice.

At first, the scientists tried to use primers that NIV had been using to detect coronaviruses in bats and other animals. However, they realized that those were not very useful in amplifying the genetic material of the coronavirus found in humans.

We had to be flexible and fast in our thinking. I am a cardiologist, that too a hard-core interventional cardiologist where split-second decisions are so very important for the life of my patients. This training has helped me tremendously in taking quick decisions, even though I may not always have been correct!

Luckily, by the second week of January 2020, a protocol for the detection of the novel coronavirus (2019-nCoV, now known as SARS-CoV-2) through RT-PCR had been prepared by a collaborative group of academic institutions in Germany and Hong Kong.[3] They had used the full genomic structure of SARS-CoV-2 published first by Chinese researchers to develop the required primers and probes. The virus's own RNA was identified as the positive control, i.e., a way of confirming that the test has indeed detected the right virus.

The ICMR had been working with a large number of academic organizations across the world for several decades. We were thus in touch with a number of them, but there were two established protocols for testing. One was the Hong Kong protocol. The other was the Berlin protocol. We adhered to those protocols immediately, and the NIV scaled up the exercise in its testing facilities. Later, two other viral research laboratories in the country got into the act with the NIV's help, which included providing them with kits, building up the infrastructure, having human resources for the viral testing and then training those people on the protocols. Some of the trainings were held during the month of March and April 2020, when we were scaling up.

The NIV team sourced the primer/probe protocols shared by the WHO on their website. NIV also procured positive controls from the Charité laboratories (Germany) and the University of Hong Kong to validate the SARS-CoV-2 real-time PCR assay. The ICMR later rolled this out across the entire country.

The NIV developed its in-house positive control[4] as well, which along with other material of the RT-PCR kit was distributed in all the laboratories engaged in COVID-19 testing nationwide.

'The tests and protocols that we developed here have become the gold standard for laboratories around the country,' Dr Varsha Potdar, who heads the National Influenza Centre at NIV, said.

HOMEMADE IS BEST

The RT-PCR test for COVID-19 involves multiple, complex steps. The first is the collection of samples using throat or nasal swabs. These swabs are kept in a special fluid called viral transport medium (VTM).

The swab goes to the laboratory, where the genetic material of the virus is separated from the sample and the transport medium, using an RNA extraction kit. Thereafter, the RT-PCR machine detects the virus using another kit.

Carrying out RT-PCR tests for large numbers of people is a logistical nightmare. We needed a constant supply of swabs, VTM, viral extraction kits and PCR kits, for use by trained personnel wearing the appropriate personal protective equipment (PPE) in quality-assured laboratories. RT-PCR tests also require handling of clinical specimens and risking infection to self.

Right at the beginning of the pandemic, India faced a dire shortage of many essential products and materials required to expand the testing. We had to import rapid testing kits and reagents needed for making quick COVID-19 diagnoses in clinical settings or in the field, as there was no domestic production. There was a shortage of PPE for health personnel, of oxygen needed for patients and even simple polyester swabs used to collect samples for testing from suspected cases.

At that point in time, we had very limited kits available in the country. Many of the kits were being imported from China. It was the largest supplier to the world; very few were available from European countries because at the time, Europe, where the number of cases was blowing up, needed the kits for itself. The US was also in a similar situation—limited kits for export. The WHO was able to supply too few to us, as it was catering to the needs of many other countries. I had a telephonic discussion with Dr Poonam Khetrapal Singh, the regional director of the WHO's South-East Asia Region. A few kits were arranged, but again, they were just a handful.

Since China was the first country that faced the challenge, it had the capacity to develop the kits. Thus, majorly, China was the only country that was supplying kits to the whole world. It was a seller's market and they could ask any price. Besides, it insisted that buyers place orders promptly, else somebody else would get the kits. We were faced with a dilemma. We needed the kits but we also had to ensure that we were not paying exorbitantly. We had a huge debate and committees were formed to discuss the matter. But we did move fast; everything was done on a war footing to decide on the price and the systems.

'At that point in time, we were literally begging for testing kits and other supplies from different parts of the world. And China, which was the major producer, would say that orders had to be placed within 12 hours or 24 hours, otherwise, it would sell to some other country,' remembers Dr Gupta.

We were trying to put in place a system. How could we suddenly order something from abroad without getting the correct quotation? Ten high-level empowered groups were created by the government. There was one group specifically assigned for testing, one for the other infrastructure. Similarly, there was one group for hospital beds and another group to deal with PPE and masks. Those days we weren't making PPE.

The government was scaling up on a war footing,[5] for which the group of Secretaries was meeting practically three or four times a week and deciding how the issues needed to be ironed out. All through, our scientific inputs were taken at every level, whether it be for the PPE, the masks, for their textile to be used or for the hospital beds to be added. Our suggestions were taken into account, including the validation of domestic kits and whether the tender had to be for seven days or 10 days, or reducing the time for the tender for getting kits from abroad. The government helped us through and through. It assisted us in setting up small scale industries and start-ups for developing kits and, initially, for transportation as well.

Dr Gupta remembers,

It was a crucial time for all of us. We had to act fast to procure testing kits to prevent the virus from spreading. It was an evening on a Saturday in March when I was driving back home from work after completing the tasks for the day, around 7.00 p.m. While I was on my way back, I got call from

Dr Bhargava to return to the office immediately. When I reached the office, I saw that he had called his full team of experts who have led disease outbreaks in the past, be it Zika virus, Nipah virus or the HIV outbreak. Our mandate was to procure as many testing kits as we could overnight. We all sat in a stuffy room till late and successfully procured some testing kits! I remember driving home late at night and coming back early to work next morning, which was a Sunday. We were truly working round the clock to make this happen.

The government leaped into action and tried its best to cut the red tape and ease the flow of imported supplies. Indian missions and embassies abroad helped identify global suppliers in a highly competitive seller's market. But we soon realized that this strategy was not sustainable. Arranging imported kits and materials was all very well in the initial phase of the pandemic response, but the enormous global competition for COVID-19-related products was making them both scarce and expensive. India would have no choice but to turn self-reliant.

TEAMWORK TRIUMPHS

In response, government agencies partnered with the domestic industry to work towards self-sufficiency in the production of rapid testing kits required in clinical settings or in the field. This kind of partnership is complex in the best of times, imagine how difficult it is in a country under lockdown. How do you get people from here to there? How do you convince airlines to carry biological material that terrifies everyone? How do you move equipment to your lab? And how on earth do you provide hands-on technical training while maintaining social distancing?

It was, in Dr Priya Abraham's words, 'A huge calling on people from different walks of life. Drivers, packers... Thousands of people were involved in the effort, and we will never know most of their names.'

Given the urgency of the situation, the government machinery also cranked up speed, facilitating smooth procurement of testing kits, setting up an inventory portal to prevent stock-outs and opting for an innovative tendering process through the Government e-Marketplace (GeM).

The strategy worked. In April 2020, the development of swabs for COVID-19 testing, for example, was locally initiated within six days and three companies were licensed to manufacture over 200,000 swabs a day and supported through grants from the Ministry of Textiles. Despite the lockdown, the production of the viral transport medium that transports clinical specimens from suspected patients was also successfully scaled up from 500,000 units per year to 500,000 units per day.

Just think about that for a moment. It doesn't exactly

fit the stereotype of slow-moving government bureaucracy, does it? The COVID-19 testing and vaccine development journey has been more like an all-out turbo-charged space mission than a Delhi rush-hour traffic jam.

After expedited approval from the government regulators, a private company developed 10 million RT-PCR tests and five million viral extraction kits. Another indigenous manufacturer developed a viral extraction kit. These testing kits needed to be validated before mass testing. Initially, these tests were validated only at NIV Pune. To expedite clearance of kits produced by the industry and reduce the burden 24 additional validation centres were approved.

'Since the start of the COVID-19 crisis our work has enabled over 5.7 million RT-PCR tests around the country,' Dr Potdar said. The team at the ICMR headquarters played a pivotal role in ensuring that testing products were delivered to the entire country, including public sector labs in every state.

To make sure the supplies reached every laboratory in a timely manner during the nationwide lockdown, the Ministry of Civil Aviation and its public and private airline partners were deployed under mission 'Lifeline UDAN'. They carried ICMR consignments of COVID-19 diagnostic materials across the country. Testing material was transported to the remotest corners of the nation like Leh, Ladakh and the Andaman and Nicobar Islands.

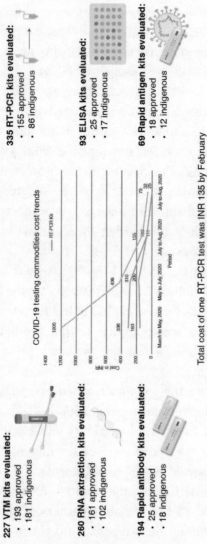

Products validated at 24 ICMR Approved Validation Centers

335 RT-PCR kits evaluated:
- 155 approved
- 86 indigenous

93 ELISA kits evaluated:
- 25 approved
- 17 indigenous

69 Rapid antigen kits evaluated:
- 18 approved
- 12 indigenous

227 VTM kits evaluated:
- 193 approved
- 181 indigenous

260 RNA extraction kits evaluated:
- 161 approved
- 102 indigenous

194 Rapid antibody kits evaluated:
- 25 approved
- 18 indigenous

COVID-19 testing commodities cost trends

RT-PCR Kit

Cost in INR

1400
1200
1000
800
600
400
200
0

1205

436

396

183

310

200

155

100

111

73

52

25

March to May, 2020   May to July, 2020   July to Aug, 2020

Period

Total cost of one RT-PCR test was INR 135 by February 2021 as compared to INR 1727 in May 2020

Figure 3.4. *A sterling example of 'Atmanirbhar Bharat'*

Doorstep deliveries were coordinated with several courier companies and state governments to reach even the most inaccessible areas. To reduce transit times, logistical complications and risks of stock outs, storage of these supplies was decentralized by building a network of 20 storage depots in a phased manner across the country.

And remember, all this happened while everyone involved was at risk of a lethal virus. For everyone involved, the work was nothing less a patriotic duty, on par with the task of defending national borders. They were prepared to sacrifice everything for the country.

4
THE GAME CHANGER

Now that we had successfully developed and produced our own testing equipment, we faced the next daunting challenge: making sure Indians everywhere had access to testing.

The scale-up of testing laboratories started with a network of 106 ICMR-funded Virus Research and Diagnostic Laboratories (VRDLs), which already had the capacity to conduct testing for viruses like SARS-CoV-2.[1]

This network of labs, many hosted by top medical colleges in the country, had been conceived soon after the outbreak of the H1N1 swine flu pandemic in 2009. The idea was to enhance the capacity for diagnosis and detection of nearly three dozen viruses of public health importance in the Indian setting.

In 2016, health policy makers prioritized expanding the network, and funding was provided to upgrade several of them to BSL-2 and BSL-3 labs. These were expected to carry out serology, RT-PCR, isolation, fluorescence microscopy, tissue culture and sequencing for all enlisted viruses. The VRDLs thus formed a solid foundation for creating testing capabilities to tackle the COVID-19 pandemic in terms of both scale and skills.

Strategically, the VRDLs served as a platform to build capacity and support new laboratories to come on board for COVID-19 testing. Beyond the VRDLs, whoever could, joined the effort: government laboratories, medical colleges and approved private laboratories. Several ICMR and non-ICMR institutes came together to begin the testing.

To ensure that no one was left behind, labs were also established in the remotest areas, such as in Ladakh, Arunachal Pradesh, Sikkim, Tripura, Mizoram, Lakshadweep and Andaman and Nicobar Islands.

The expansion of COVID-19 testing infrastructure was greatly helped by the participation of the private enterprise. The key role in roping them into the national effort was played by a government agency, the National Accreditation Board for Testing and Calibration Laboratories (NABL).

The NABL provided oversight to ensure that only qualified labs were made testing centres. There is no official data or register of the more than 200,000 private labs in India, which are also of highly uneven quality. The costs for various diagnostic tests are also not uniform across such labs.

Given the rapidly growing demand for testing facilities, the NABL adopted novel ways to inspect and certify potential labs amidst the national lockdown, including virtual tours. By the end of July 2020, more than 400 private sector laboratories had successfully come on board for testing.

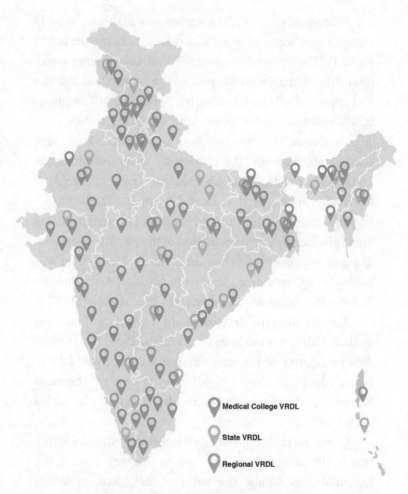

Medical College VRDL

State VRDL

Regional VRDL

*Figure 4.1: Network of Virus Research and
Diagnostic Laboratories (VRDLs) in India*

One of the important consequences of expanding the number of laboratories available and also producing the materials needed within the country, was a sharp drop in the costs of testing. The total cost of one RT-PCR test in early 2021 had come down to just ₹135, as compared to ₹1,727 in March 2020.

'It is a big achievement for India to have become self-sufficient and scaled up its COVID-19 testing capacity,' observed Dr Soumya Swaminathan, chief scientist, WHO. According to her, it was the result of the government of India taking the pandemic extremely seriously and putting in place the appropriate measures needed, right from the beginning of the outbreak.

GETTING IT RIGHT

Setting up a laboratory with quality testing and safety standards involves a four-step process:

1. Ensuring the availability of proper infrastructure as per WHO guidelines; this includes a cabinet to ensure safety from the virus
2. Reviewing the documentation using photo and video evidence
3. Training the staff at a VRDL
4. Conducting a trial run to ensure independent functioning of the laboratory

To hasten the operationalization of the network of COVID-19 testing laboratories, we set up 14 Centres of Excellence in different medical institutes to guide new testing sites through those four steps. These centres mentored government and private medical colleges in their catchment areas and created a molecular virology laboratory network in a remarkably short time.[2]

To further ensure high-quality testing, an inter-laboratory quality control programme was set up. This network linked the rapidly growing network of RT-PCR labs to 38 regional quality control labs. They were in turn connected to NIV Pune, which was designated a Global Reference Lab for COVID-19 by the WHO.

Scientists at the NIV and the ICMR helped train staff in all the laboratories across India through dozens of virtual conferencing sessions. We anticipated a big demand for testing and undertook training sessions on a war footing. Many sessions lasted through the night. Thousands of virtual trainings were conducted by the ICMR, including refresher trainings for testing and data collection. In fact, even before our testing portal went online, the ICMR staff was manually entering data on the portal. Once the portal went live, it became the biggest in the world.

In the process of fighting the pandemic, we also reached a new level of technological prowess much sooner than we would have otherwise. It is a heartening side-effect of the immense efforts and innovative spirit of everyone who worked on the response.

NEW WINE, OLD BOTTLE

The RT-PCR technique was one of the first, and later the most common, methods for COVID-19 testing. But we used many other processes as well. In some cases, we repurposed testing platforms originally used for other infectious diseases. Consider TrueNAT, for one.[3]

TrueNAT is an indigenous test platform, developed in 2018, for detecting tuberculosis (especially multidrug-resistant TB). In May 2020, we rejigged it for COVID-19. TrueNAT, which detects genetic material from the virus, involves minimal risk of infection and contamination. This meant that district hospitals across the country could also use it, unlike the RT-PCR, whose use was limited to well-equipped hospitals and laboratories.

TrueNAT platforms are light and portable, so teams could set up mobile testing centres or kiosks in containment zones, instead of having to transport samples to labs. It is also speedy—clinical specimens can go from RNA extraction to amplification in less than 60 minutes. This helped immensely in confirming cases, contact tracing, isolation and clinical management.

By the end of 2020, as many as 2,530 workstations based on TrueNAT technology were operational at 1,008 sites in 530 districts across India.[4] Several other countries emulated India's pioneering work on repurposing TB diagnostic equipment for COVID-19 testing. One such example is the COVID Nudge used in the United Kingdom (UK).

To increase testing capacity, the ICMR also pressed several high-throughput platforms, also originally meant for TB testing, into service. In June 2020, we modified three state-of-the-art Cobas 6800/8800 platforms; capable of handling 1,400–4,000 samples per day, and added them to the national network. This meant a dozen more labs, and reduced turnaround time and exposure to infection.

Even as we were working within the country to ramp up testing, there was an external challenge before us: to help our people stranded abroad due to the pandemic.

THE IRAN RESCUE MISSION

The ancient Iranian city of Qom is famous worldwide for its intricately woven carpets. They are known for their fine quality and dense knotting, sometimes up to 240,000–1,600,000 knots per sq.m. carpet.

Legend has it that the artisans of Qom deliberately leave a small flaw in their carpets, as making them perfect would be considered an attempt to 'challenge God'!

In early 2020 though, it was the Maker Himself who challenged Qom's residents as the COVID-19 pandemic swept through the population causing untold misery. It also left stranded in its wake thousands of Indian pilgrims visiting holy sites in the city at the time.

Coming to the stranded pilgrims' rescue, in one of the most inspiring missions carried out during the entire pandemic period, were scientists from NIV Pune. As the Indian embassy in Tehran was flooded with calls for help, the Indian government and the ICMR organized a team to fly in and help the pilgrims come home.

While arranging for them to be flown back to India was not a problem per se, we had to screen them for COVID-19 first. The Iranian authorities, overwhelmed by the upsurge in domestic cases, did not have the wherewithal to carry out these tests. New Delhi moved swiftly to fill the gap.

'The call came out of the blue, informing me that I had to pack up and leave for Tehran within a few days,' Dr Gururaj Deshpande, a scientist at NIV and member of a small team of two scientists and two engineers picked for the mission, recalled. They flew to Iran, in the twenty-first century equivalent of a magic carpet from Qom.

The team was mandated to set up an RT-PCR testing facility in Iran to collect swab samples from five cities in Iran and send them back to India. Those who tested positive for COVID-19 would be put in quarantine before being allowed to travel.

'I was deeply concerned about the risk our scientists

were taking by going to Iran at a time when there was so little known about the pandemic and when there was so much fear,' Dr Priya Abraham said. However, the mission was a top national priority, and for Dr Deshpande and his team, it was a patriotic duty they willingly performed. It was also an adventure, despite the risks.

Once in Iran, the team went about quickly setting up a site with all safety protocols in place to receive Indians willing to get the tests done, document them and provide advice on what to do if they tested positive. There were many challenges, not all of them medical. For example, residents near the testing facility set up by the Indian scientists, objected to its presence, fearful of COVID-19 spreading in their neighbourhood. The site had to be shifted to the basement of the Indian embassy in Tehran to continue with the operations smoothly.

The Indian embassy also established a quarantine centre to house more than 250 Indians infected with the coronavirus, the largest such facility for Indians anywhere outside India at that time. More than 2,000 Indians made it safely back home. A total of 308 samples tested positive for SARS-CoV-2 and those people were put in quarantine before being allowed to travel home.

These enthusiastic young ICMR scientists had the typical spirit of so many involved in the COVID-19 enterprise: bravery, efficiency, intelligence, enthusiasm and compassion.

My role basically was to request the scientists of ICMR-NIV and the NIV director to urgently deploy our team to Iran. You can imagine the kind of fear that the families of the people chosen to go to Iran had nurtured. There was also the logistics of sending the team quickly. Passports were prepared in Delhi in double quick time, and visa was arranged within a few hours! The team left the very next day. There was a war being waged on the virus, and we could not lose time.

The members went in batches of one or two, sharing the equipment that went with them. After they came back, with the mission successful, they were isolated at the ICMR-NIV guest house, which was used as a bubble. They stayed in that bubble and completed the 10-day quarantine.

RAPID ANTIGEN TESTS

Meanwhile, the national task force discussed the issue of rapid antigen tests threadbare. The rapid tests had become absolutely necessary, as we had big wave in June 2020 in Delhi. It was no easy task. We had limited number of qualified labs in March–April. Besides, many times, the samples had to be flown in from different parts of the country, to the high-throughput laboratories. They were tested and the reports were given on the third day.

Once the first wave came to Delhi, we were flooded

with a huge number of tests to be done. We decided to take up the rapid antigen tests on a big scale and get them validated immediately. We found the test's sensitivity to be about 60 to 70 per cent.

We developed an algorithm in June 2020 clearly stating that if the test was positive in someone symptomatic, they would be considered case of COVID-19. If they were negative and symptomatic, then they would need to do an RT-PCR test.[5] The WHO recognized the rapid antigen tests in September. Thereafter, the tests that we were conducting in India became a routine in different parts of the world. They were also being used in South Korea at that point in time.

India became one of the first countries in the world to validate and include rapid antigen testing for COVID-19 diagnosis, in mid-2020. 'Antigen' is a fancy word for a toxic material; in this case, the SARS-CoV-2 virus. These tests work by detecting the 'spike protein' on the surface of the coronavirus that lets it enter the human cell and elicits the body's immune response.

The easily portable POC diagnostic tests, capable of giving results in just 30 minutes, proved to be extremely useful in certain settings like containment zones where quick results were required. It provided the much-needed impetus to the government's strategy of 'test, track and treat'.

Antigen testing does not amplify the genetic material

in samples, therefore, at times, there is not enough antigen material to be detectable. This results in false negative tests, making them somewhat unreliable and requiring confirmation through a regular RT-PCR test, particularly when someone is symptomatic but tests negative with the rapid antigen test. Positive tests in a symptomatic individual don't require confirmation.

Currently, the RT-PCR and rapid antigen tests account for most of the COVID-19 tests in India, with part of the burden shared by repurposed platforms like TrueNAT.

Detect immune repsonse to SARS-CoV-2 exposure

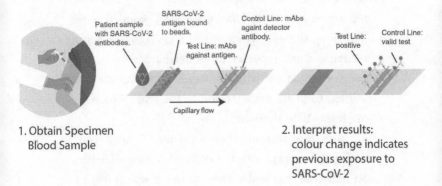

1. Obtain Specimen
   Blood Sample

2. Interpret results:
   colour change indicates previous exposure to SARS-CoV-2

Figure 4.2: Antibody tests for confirming COVID-19 infection

VIRUS VERSUS VISION

My colleague, Dr Sanghamitra Pati, director, ICMR-Regional Medical Research Centre (RMRC), Bhubaneswar narrated a remarkable anecdote that I would like to share here, verbatim, to emphasize the urgent need for development of a rapid antigen test kit.

> I vividly remember the date, 25 April 2020, late evening, around 9.00 p.m. A text message flashed on my mobile: 'Something urgent to discuss; can I speak to you now?' I replied in the affirmative in a flash. The SOS was from Dr Manmath Das, a young energetic retina surgeon in Bhubaneswar city. *'What could be the urgency for an ophthalmologist?'* I wondered. At that time, the eye symptoms of COVID were being recognized and reported by clinicians. Maybe he too had seen a patient with unilateral conjunctivitis and wanted to bring my attention to the issue. That was my immediate thought.
>
> In a few seconds, he called me. 'I need your advice on a very critical matter. A young diabetic, 30 years old, has just arrived at our hospital from a small town 120 kilometres away, with 2.5 hours' road journey. He is a known case of diabetic retinopathy; with complete loss of vision in the right eye. For the past one year, he is ambulatory with his left eye.

Today, he had a sudden drop in vision in the left eye, and thankfully, has reached us by arranging transport as early as possible for him. It appears to be complete retinal detachment. I have to operate on him by tomorrow morning anyhow, else it might be too late. However, I don't know if he has novel coronavirus or not. As you know, we have limited RT-PCR testing now. Your lab is the only one in the city now. By the time the reports come, it might be too late to save his vision. Many of my acquaintances are cautioning me not to take the risk, as I don't know his exposure status. Further, I have two small kids and aged parents at home. My father is being treated for a long-term debilitating illness too. On the other hand, if I don't do the surgery tomorrow, this person will be losing vision forever. I have to save his left eye anyhow. He is young, has a long life to look forward to, it's a matter of his whole life and future as well. But if I go for his surgery, I might stand all the potential risks of getting infected. Please guide.'

Dr Das was obviously in a dilemma. The genuine concern in his voice was resonating with appeal and commitment to his patient's wellbeing. I could well realize the apprehension of a young ophthalmologist with small children and aged ailing parents. He was caught in a bind between the restoration of vision for his patient and the fear of an invisible unknown virus infecting him. Here, the surgeon wanted my guidance.

I weighed his own risk with the benefit to a patient's future vision. But there was not much time to think. I quickly checked the case load of the block from where the patient hailed. Thankfully it was a green zone. Then I asked a few questions like whether the patient or his family member or their vehicle driver had any symptoms. He responded in the negative.

'Then take all possible precautionary measures (with goggles and N-95, protective wear) for yourself and the patient, and go ahead with the surgery,' I said, and added, 'After the surgery, watch the patient and you too remain in isolation for 5–7 days.' I told him that if the patient showed no symptoms, he could return to his village, and the doctor could go home. We had to then quickly arrange all the necessary protective gears and the surgery was done as per schedule, the next morning. The patient was discharged after four days. Dr Das remained in isolation as per protocol and went back home uneventfully.

No one can feel such emotionally charged moments unless they themselves have gone through them. On that day, we both subconsciously perceived the need for some way to rule out a patient as

COVID-19 positive at the point of care. I am sure, many patients and physicians must have faced such dilemmatic moments alike at that time.

The ICMR had thought of it too in foresight. Because, after six weeks, in mid-June, it announced the launch of the validated rapid antigen testing kit. The rest is history. This POC testing kit was bolstered by a stringent validation accompanied with a very simple yet rigorous algorithm. From the third week of June onwards, the state started procuring the kits in lots. All hospitals were given due ID and password to perform rapid antigen testing with linking to a nearby RT-PCR Lab. It was a true game-changer in the COVID-19 testing race against time.

In August 2020, I got a call from Dr Das again. This time he sounded excited. 'Do you remember the patient I operated on? Today he had come for his follow-up, and his left eye vision is almost back to normal. Now he can lead a normal life. I feel so contented that I took the right decision and sought your support at the right moment. The situation is so much better now, thanks to the ICMR's rapid antigen testing roll-out. We don't face problems as before. The rapid antigen test is done at the entry to the hospital itself and asymptomatic negative patients are immediately transferred to the respective units. Thus, the triaging for non-

COVID patients is eased out with expedited access to treatment.'

I felt so happy. Countless lives must have been saved thanks to this timely in-sight.

5
WHY RESEARCH MATTERS

very October, in the northeast-Indian state of Nagaland, members of the ethnic Bomrr clan of the Yimchunger tribe carry out a special harvest that they have practised for over seven generations.

Climbing up a cliff, the Bomrr stack firewood at the openings of the caves and light a firelight a fire to produce large plumes of smoke. Their targets are the thousands of bats that live in those caves. The bats either fall dead inside or are struck down with sticks as they fly out. They are cooked as a delicacy or dried and stored for future use.

Given that bats are known to be reservoirs of a number of deadly pathogens, including coronaviruses and filoviruses, an international team with Indian researchers carried out a study of the Bomrr tribe in 2018. The researchers collected blood samples from the bat hunters, who are exposed to saliva, blood and excreta from the bat species *Rousettus leschenaultii* and *Eonycteris spelaea*. Samples of the bats were also collected. The study presented the first evidence of a spill-over disease that goes from wildlife to humans, in this case filoviruses from bats infecting people.[1]

The ICMR has been carrying out research on bat behaviour and ecology since 2001, an area of study that is relatively new in India. The NIV's bat surveillance team, the only one of its kind in the country, has been carrying out a mapping exercise all over India to get a clearer picture of the distribution and abundance, as well as proximity of humans to bat species that are also carriers of various potentially dangerous viruses.

Following the advent of the COVID-19 pandemic, the NIV's bat surveillance unit carried out a study to assess the presence of coronaviruses in the Indian Flying Fox and Rousettus species of bats found in different parts of India.[2] Using RT-PCR tests, the study found pathogenic coronaviruses in the two species.

The world of medical research is unique. A study that proves that a particular line of treatment does *not* work is considered as important as finding a cure. Why is this? Because ruling out unproven therapies are important to avoid wasting time, resources and lives.

As medical professionals worldwide searched for possible treatments to help those severely affected by COVID-19, one option that briefly created quite a buzz early on was plasma therapy.[3] This involved the transfusion of blood plasma from recovered patients—also known as convalescent plasma—to those currently infected in the hope that the antibodies from the former would benefit the latter.

Plasma therapy has been used over the last hundred years for many diseases, but never has anyone conclusively seen whether the treatment benefits or harms. COVID-19 brought to the fore the demand for plasma therapy once more. We could not ignore it, since patients and their relatives insisted on it as a form of treatment in desperation. The demand even led to black-marketing of the plasma! Besides, we as doctors felt that if we did not try the therapy out, we might potentially lose a life.

To understand whether convalescent plasma therapy really did benefit patients, the ICMR carried out the PLACID trial from April to July 2020, with over 464 participants with confirmed moderate COVID-19. The study was conducted across 39 public/private hospitals in record time and was the largest such exercise of its kind anywhere in the world.[4]

The results finally showed that convalescent plasma had no effect. The trial had major implications for treatment protocols around the world and was a valuable contribution to the global understanding of COVID-19 therapeutics. Like the WHO Solidarity trial,[5] [6] where the Indian component was coordinated by the ICMR-National AIDS Research Institute (NARI),[7] and several other trials, the PLACID trial too demonstrated what not to rely on—as valuable an insight as knowing what to rely on.

The PLACID trial was outstanding in terms of pace and the scientific methodology followed. Usually, such trials in India take several years to materialize. But if this pandemic has taught my colleagues and me one thing, it is that we can operate at double or triple the normal speed and still maintain high quality. The amount of time taken for clinical trials in the pre-pandemic era was long. PLACID trials were expedited and were done in a real-world setting. Incidentally, there still are several sites which have not taken funds from the ICMR team for conducting the trial.

Apart from its scientific merit and public health significance, the trial was also one of the few studies that was completely indigenous in design, implementation, analysis and policy uptake. The trial showed India's capacity for generating medical evidence on a large scale, in the middle of an evolving pandemic.

DEMOCRATIZATION OF RESEARCH

We chose to study convalescent plasma because, unlike all other new treatments which were in uncertain supply, this could be the most easily available therapy.

Our team of researchers put together a study protocol with help from haematologists, transfusion medicine specialists and internists. Once the protocol was ready, our instinct was to implement it at a few centres of repute. But there were major concerns. Would it be equitable to restrict clinical trials, an important vehicle for providing access to treatment, to a few hospitals? Would it represent the reality of India, which encompasses both metropolitan cities and rural villages?

Bearing these questions in mind, we opened our recruitment to every hospital that had the requisite infrastructure, and agreed to provide free treatment to trial participants. The response was overwhelming. Despite having busy clinical schedules, doctors on the frontline were keen to participate, and more than 100 hospitals responded to our call. Eventually, despite their tight budgets, over three dozen hospitals would enrol several hundred patients in just three months. The journey to get to that point, however, was not easy, as Dr Aparna Mukherjee, the principal investigator of the trial remembers.

The first hurdle: how to set up multidisciplinary teams at every site, with a clinician, a transfusion medicine specialist and a microbiologist—all of whom were already overwhelmed with working in under-staffed settings, while donning perspiration-drenched PPE?

However, the sites did manage to get these teams together. As it turned out, the sites which performed best were not the ones that had the best infrastructure or prior experience in research, but those that put together the most coordinated teams.

As the cases of COVID-19 were still rising, the country was under a lockdown and people were generally avoiding hospitals, getting plasma donors to hospitals was a challenge. The sites, however, put in exemplary efforts to collect plasma. Each site called hundreds of potential donors, arranged cars for pick-up and drop off and designed innovative information campaigns to get plasma.

The biggest hurdle for the central team was assuring data quality. To this end, we carried out multiple training sessions to discuss the protocol and fill in the electronic data capture forms. All the investigators met online weekly, and we also connected with individual investigators twice every week. Most importantly, to assure quality, the central team focused on fostering relationships with all the investigators. This helped create an environment conducive to discuss the challenges faced by investigators and find solutions, rather than indulge in the blame-game culture of finding faults. These relationships bore fruit, as site investigators took ownership of the trial.

The goal of research is to generate knowledge through hard data. Conducting this trial taught us that successful high-quality, large-scale trials are rooted in capacity building, training and having respect for local health systems. We learnt that, as in other areas of life, generating evidence is also best done by fostering trustworthy relationships—with effective communication, clear ownership and teamwork at their core.

RESEARCH DURING LOCKDOWN

Imagine having to solve a complicated jigsaw puzzle where the pieces are all in different rooms and on different floors, the stairs are broken and you must find your way around blindfolded, and then put the pieces together as fast as possible before the whole house falls down. If this sounds difficult, just imagine trying to understand, isolate and work out how to treat a mysterious virus during an international lockdown.

Researchers typically came to work early in the morning and went home very late—if they managed to go home at all. At the ICMR headquarters in New Delhi too, key staff members often worked till 2.00 a.m., which also meant long hours for everyone else, from security guards to those running the cafeteria. Virtual boardroom meetings at the oddest hours became the norm. To further complicate logistics, the national lockdown affected everything. Guesthouses were full of scientists, most of whom were women, who had the added worry of families at home to think about. On the one hand, home with older parents and young children; on the other, a high-security lab with a deadly virus to contain.

The research got a boost, particularly since there was already a system in place in an organization that is more than 111 years old. This is a system in which thinking is very scientific from the very beginning and there is some sense of hierarchy. This was very good, and could be leveraged at that point in time, particularly in the warlike situation of the pandemic. I think it worked best for India. It was our work culture which helped us tremendously during those hours of crisis.

Scientific arguments were always welcome and encouraged, but at the same time, there was a sense of discipline, which really led to achieving what we have— whether it be my video conferencing with all the directors, the directors with their scientists and the scientists with their technical officers. It was woven together exceptionally, whether it be the different institutes working together, different labs working together or scientists working together—for the larger good of the country.

While everyone involved made terrific sacrifices and risked their own safety to work during a pandemic,[8] women, whether they were scientists, transport personnel, bureaucrats, health workers or whatever else, had the added burden of facing the challenges of COVID-19 as well as managing households, children who were home, elder care and transportation to and from work in uncertain times. With all that, they shone, and retained their enthusiasm for the job, and for science. '75 per cent of my team were women,' Dr Priya Abraham proudly stated. Women were indeed the real superheroes of the entire effort.

Dr Abraham is the perfect role model for young people, especially young women, to get excited about careers in science. If she weren't so busy managing a passionate team of scientists and saving the world from COVID-19, she could be a wonderful STEM brand ambassador.

I had to deal with all kinds of people at every level: within the institutes, within ICMR, within the scientific agencies of the country, other public health agencies or medical colleges and even the press and the bureaucracy. We had a list of about 570 different treatments which had been proposed by people. This included one involving a locket with a stone in it that produced chlorine. We faced enormous pressure. There were people who had their own companies and wanted to do certain things which were not working that well or wanted to know whether their ideas were working. But we knew we had to put our scientific resources in the targeted direction, remain undistracted from these unproven, non-scientific cures.

REPURPOSING INFRASTRUCTURE

During the pandemic, the strengths and capacities at all the ICMR institutes and other facilities were pooled together to get the best possible outputs. Repurposing helped us manage many things.

The staff was engaged in a series of activities like sero-surveys, follow-up of vaccine rollouts, testing, validation of diagnostic commodities, creating depots for storage, distribution of commodities, coordination with states,

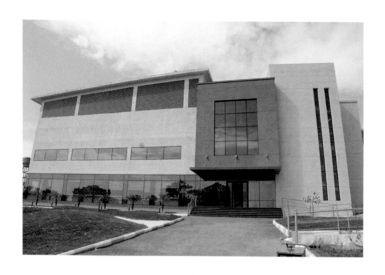

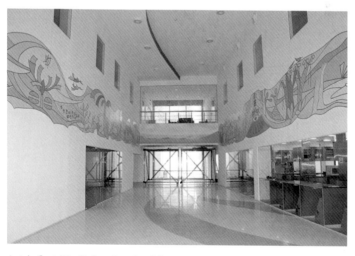

Asia's first Bio Safety Level-4 laboratory at ICMR-NIV, Pune played a pivotal role in tackling the outbreak of COVID-19

Source: ICMR

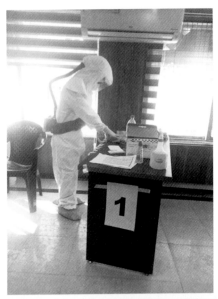

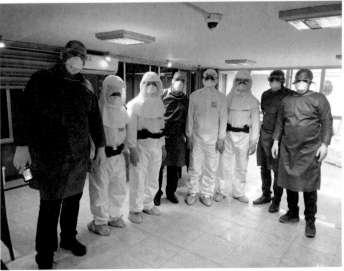

Laboratory established in Iran to help stranded citizens to get tested and brought back home

Source: ICMR

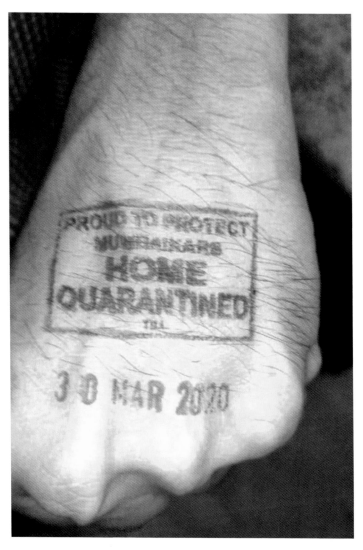

Stamping: Measure to limit the spread of COVID-19
Source: Special Arrangement, published in The Hindu

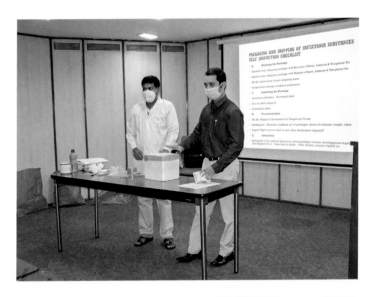

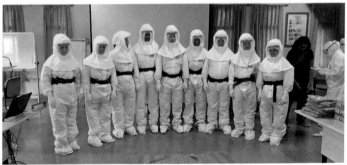

Stringent training on Biosafety and Biosecurity at ICMR institutes

Source: ICMR

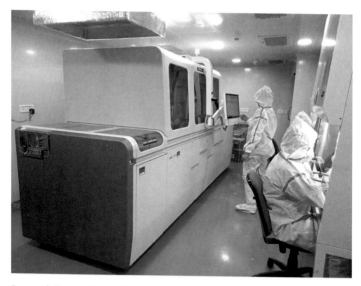

State-of-the-art High-Throughput COVID-19 testing machine (Cobas 6800) deployed at 10 places nationwide
Source: ICMR

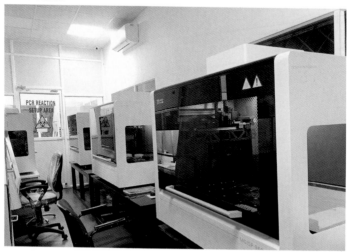

Mega RT-PCR laboratory at Noida with a capacity to conduct 10,000 COVID-19 tests per day
Source: ICMR

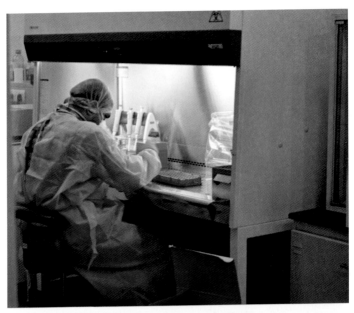

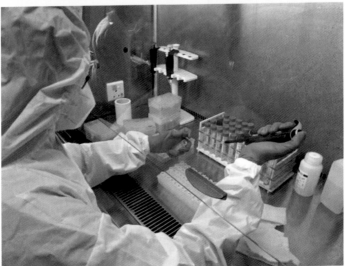

Sample processing and setting up of RT-PCR tests
Source: ICMR

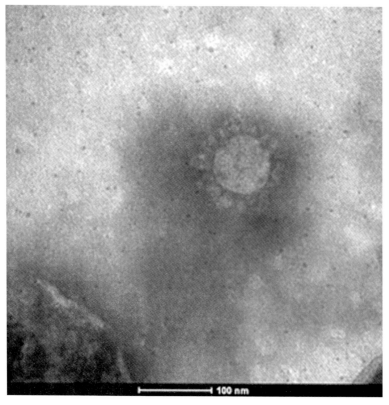

First isolation and imaging of SARS-Cov-2; India was fifth in the world to achieve this feat

Source: ICMR

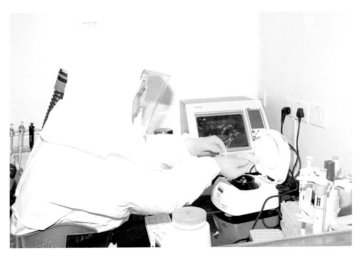

Scientist working in Bio Safety Level-4 conditions handling SARS-CoV-2
Source: ICMR

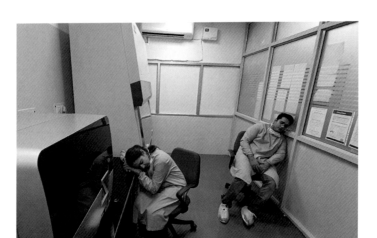

Exhausted laboratory staff after working non-stop for 16 hours
Source: ICMR

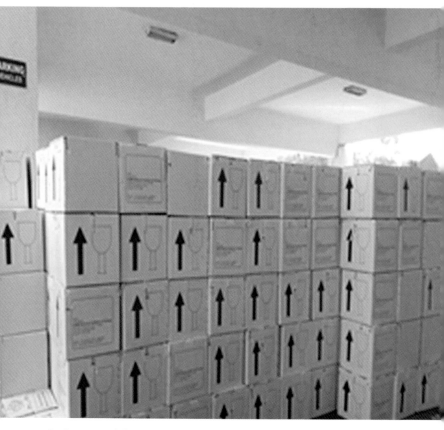

Packaging and shipment of diagnostic reagents to other centres
Source: ICMR

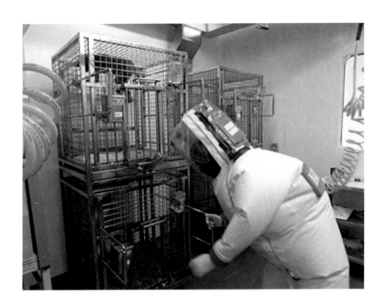

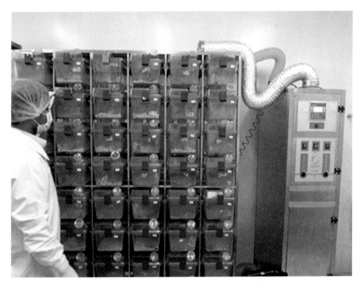

ICMR-NIV's BSL-4 highly equipped for Covaxin animal studies
Source: ICMR

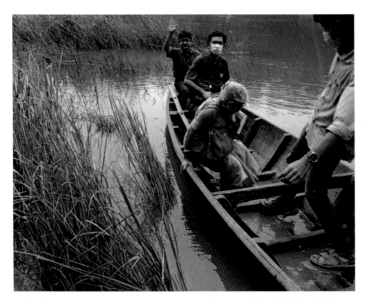

COVID-19 national sero-survey team from ICMR-NICED, Kolkata, travelling by boat to collect samples after the bridge collapsed due to Cyclone Amphan

Source: ICMR

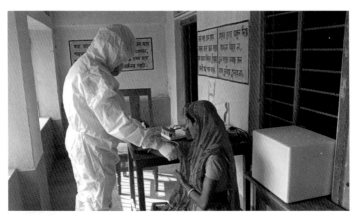

Reaching the nooks and corners of the country for national sero-survey for COVID-19

Source: ICMR

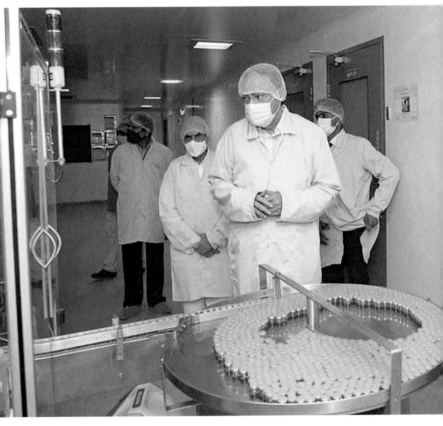

Honourable Vice President M. Venkaiah Naidu visiting the BBIL Facility, Hyderabad

Source: Bharat Biotech/ Twitter

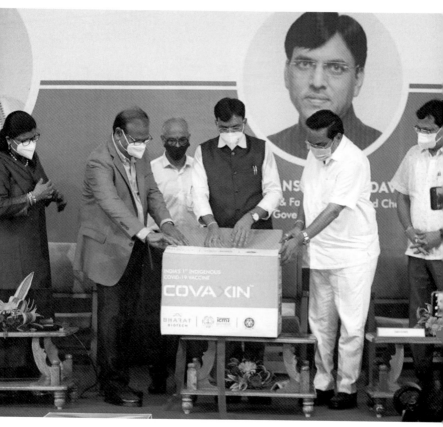

Honourable Minister of Health and Family Welfare, Dr Mansukh Mandaviya launching the first commercial batch of Covaxin manufactured at the Gujarat facility

Source: Bharat Biotech/Twitter

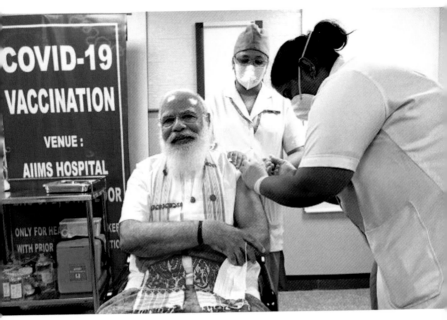

When the turn came for people above 60, Honourable Prime Minister Narendra Modi received his first dose of Covaxin

Source: PIB

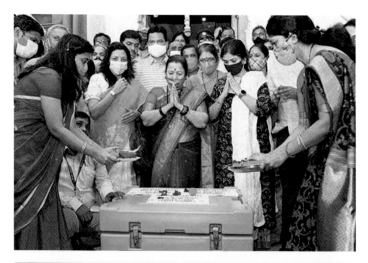

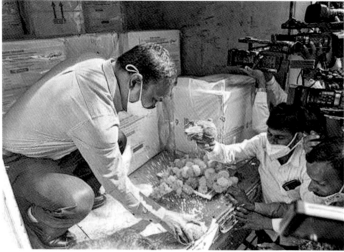

COVID-19 vaccines receive a traditional welcome
Source: PTI

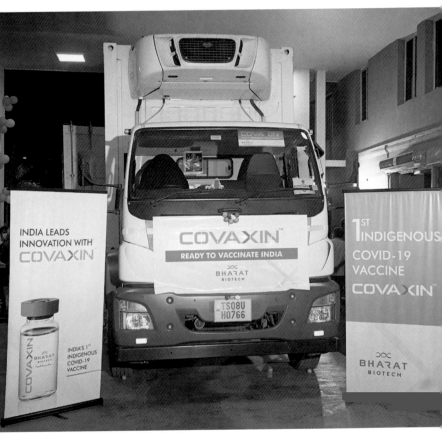

(Above and facing page) First batch of Covaxin being dispatched

Source: Bharat Biotech

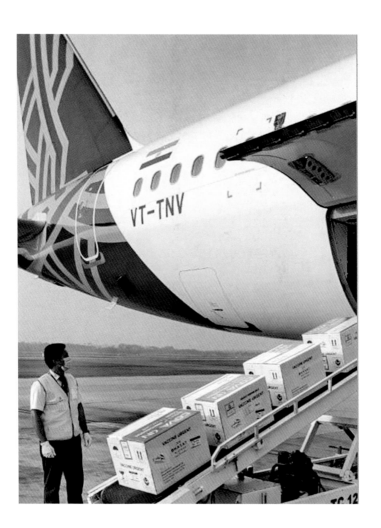

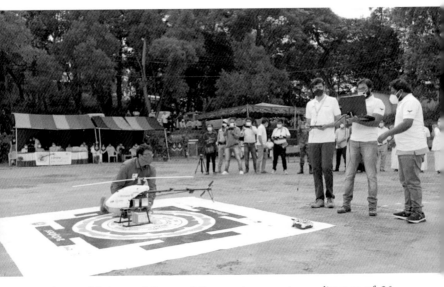

Successful drone delivery of the vaccine covering a distance of 26 kilometres from Bishnupur District Hospital to Karang Island in Manipur. It crossed the famous Loktak Lake. India became the first country in South Asia to achieve this feat

Source: ICMR

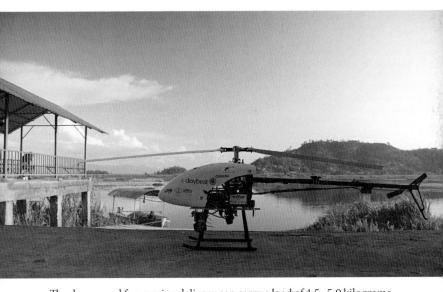

The drone used for vaccine delivery can carry a load of 4.5–5.0 kilograms approximately, which is around 900 doses at a time

Source: ICMR

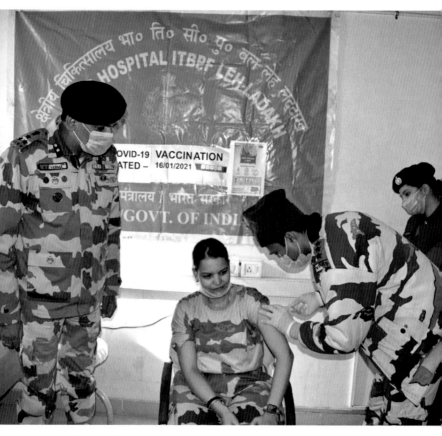

Frontline workers receiving their first dose in January, 2021
Source: ITBP/ Twitter

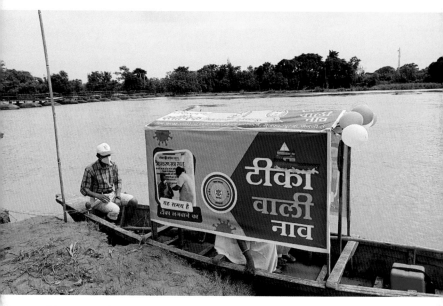

Vaccination boats: Custom solutions to reach flooded regions of Assam

Source: MoHFW/ Twitter

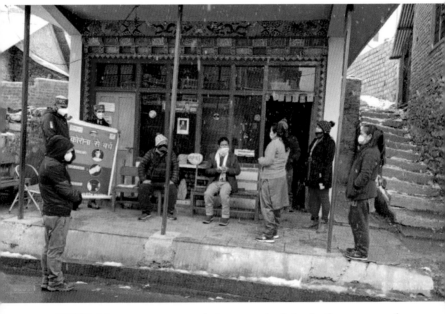

COVID-19 awareness camp being organized in far-flung areas of Lahaul-Spiti, Himachal Pradesh (11,000 feet above sea level) by the ICMR-Keylong Field Unit team

Source : ICMR

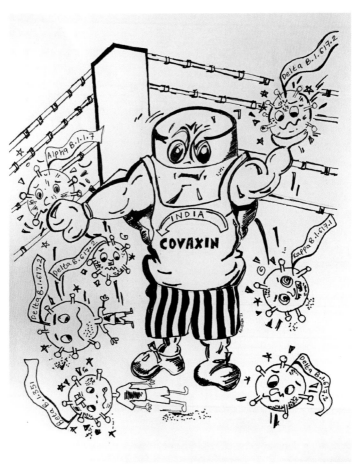

Doodle showing efficacy of Covaxin over different variants of concern
Photo Credit: Anushka Kalaskar, a student of MSc Virology at ICMR-NIV
Source : ICMR

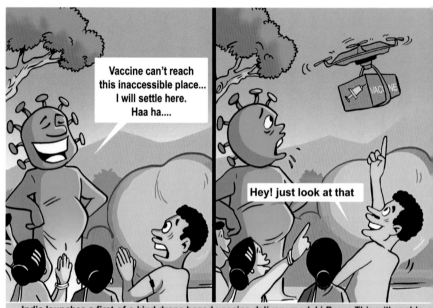

A cartoon depicting the effect of drone delivery of vaccines in difficult-to-reach areas

Source : PIB Bhubaneswar

etc. It wasn't business as usual, as we pivoted from our routine ongoing work and research to various institutes, labs and outreach units to deal with an unprecedented new situation. We leveraged our capacities holistically and it definitely paid off!

During the pandemic, the ICMR institutes also perfected the art of multitasking. This has again hugely benefited the entire system and helped the ICMR family fight the pandemic in unison. The sero-survey was done by all the different institutes, whether it be the nutrition institute or the regional medical research centre in Gorakhpur or a cancer centre or a tuberculosis institute. They all got into the Covid framework of mind. And they were all involved in fighting Covid in every which way, whether it be data collection, serum sample collection,[9] testing or development and distribution of testing kits or even small animal studies.

One example of such innovations was the setting up of a high-throughput laboratory at our institute in Noida. We had a building with a defunct incinerator in the animal house of the institute. In April 2020, the incinerator was removed and the whole building was repurposed as a high-throughput laboratory, with more than 12 RT-PCR machines, having a capacity of up to 4,000 tests per day. Initially samples were flown in here from different parts of the country to be tested rapidly. Technology played a great role. Today, we have labs in nearly every district of

India, and that is reassuring.

Another big step forward was strengthening our field epidemiological capacities. India has been a torchbearer in conducting repeated nationwide sero-surveys for SARS-CoV-2. These field epidemiological capacities are expected to be repurposed for several other important studies, particularly to determine the burden of vaccine-preventable diseases and assessing post-vaccination trends.

Nurturing the country's laboratory infrastructure[10] has been another important outcome, from a long-term health systems perspective. We all felt the need to establish molecular diagnostic capacities for detecting infectious disease pathogens.

'Earlier we had only a few labs in the country that had the people and facilities to diagnose and study viral disease outbreaks. But now there is a good quality lab in virtually every district of India,' Dr Samiran Panda, head, ICMR's Epidemiology and Communicable Diseases Division said.

This is a tremendous value addition to India's public health system. We are determined to effectively repurpose our infrastructure and human capital (read: all the dedicated people involved in this work and future scientists) for other infectious diseases like tuberculosis, respiratory viral infections including influenza and other emerging/re-emerging infections and zoonotic infections.

The backbone of health infrastructure in the country has been a socialistic public health-, medical college- and district hospital-based infrastructure. We have the same system for research. These can all be renovated. They can be repaired. They can be repurposed for COVID-19, as we have done for the ICMR institutes and demonstrated how we repaired our infrastructure, not only during the pandemic but before the pandemic also. The repurpose can be done for testing, research, patient care, etc. We wrote down the ideas as they occurred to us. Even simple things, like better toilet facilities in hospitals, tackling the stray menace in hospital premises, wall posters falling off, etc., were noted down.

Covid gave us an opportunity to revisit these issues and fix them. In the long term, as I have mentioned earlier, we need to spend more on healthcare. There are countries such as the US which spend 20 per cent of their $20 trillion budget on healthcare. We've been spending only one per cent, although that is being increased now. We are targeting healthcare spending to 2.5 per cent of the GDP and the government is moving in this direction rapidly.

ICMR'S REGIONAL RESEARCH INITIATIVE

India and the ICMR's initiative to work together with and support other countries in the region on the vaccine front is not new. A year after the deadly outbreak of the Nipah virus disease in Kerala in 2018, the ICMR helped launch a new platform called 'Regional Enabler for the South East

Asia Research Collaboration for Health' or RESEARCH, to find solutions to emerging and re-emerging infectious diseases in the WHO's South-East Asia Region in August 2019.

Over the last decade and a half, the region has been home to a host of emerging infectious diseases, which have taken a heavy toll on human and animal populations as well as national economies. The region has witnessed outbreaks of many of the nine most serious infectious threats identified by the WHO globally, including Crimean-Congo haemorrhagic fever (CCHF), Middle East respiratory syndrome coronavirus (MERS-CoV), severe acute respiratory syndrome (SARS) and Zika virus disease.

The new research platform is meant to pool together resources at the regional level to help deal with various aspects of these outbreaks. The goal is to conduct multi-country clinical trials, epidemiological and clinical research studies that will make a difference to all of us.

6

AN INDIAN VACCINE: FROM DREAM TO ROLL-OUT

L egend has it that Edward Jenner, the eighteenth-century British scientist, discovered the vaccine for smallpox because of an incident that took place when he was in his early teens. Apparently, as a 13-year-old boy, he overheard a beautiful milkmaid boast that her flawless complexion was because she had cowpox, a disease caused by virus found in cattle.[1]

The cowpox, according to her, protected her from smallpox and prevented her from getting an ugly pockmarked face. This was the hypothesis that Jenner would later test and confirm, leading to the vaccine for smallpox, a disease that had been the scourge of humanity for millennia. Not surprisingly, the term 'vaccine' that Jenner used, comes from the Latin word *vacca*, which means cow.

Vaccination is inarguably one of humanity's greatest innovations. It is the most significant pharmaceutical intervention for the prevention of any infectious disease. It is no exaggeration to say that vaccination can, and has, changed the course of generations and civilizations.

Vaccines have helped not just control but even completely wipe out diseases that have held humanity hostage for millennia. Apart from smallpox—the dragon that was finally slain worldwide in 1980—vaccines also helped halt the spread and impact of diseases such as measles, mumps, diphtheria, tetanus and polio in most countries around the world.

While everyone knew that a vaccine was essential to stop COVID-19, nobody believed it would take less than (at least) two years to develop one. Before this, the shortest time for producing a vaccine was four years— for mumps.[2]

However, as COVID-19 wreaked havoc by disrupting health systems and disrupting economies across the globe, the world put in an unprecedented effort to develop both treatments and vaccines. These are desperate times. We are living through a moment that future generations will read about in their history books and certainly in their medical textbooks.

Scientists in research labs across the globe raced against time to work on innovative solutions using new technologies or products, some of them repurposed from other uses. Vaccine development was speeded up by combining what we already knew about coronaviruses, such as previous research done on the SARS and MERS viruses. We also tapped our accumulated know-how on RNA vaccines.

With the SARS-CoV-2 virus finally isolated, cultured and better understood, we at the ICMR started thinking seriously about developing a vaccine of our own. The global and national situations were dire; it was clearly time for bold action.

It is important to remember that while COVID-19 is new, we were not completely starting from scratch. We had seen coronaviruses before and had worked on vaccines before. This prior experience was an excellent foundation.

Apart from hard science, vaccine development also requires manufacturing power and a whole lot of logistical maneuvering. The average time from discovery to production for any vaccine in the past was 10 years. We were on the lookout for industrial partners with whom we could collaborate for a vaccine. The first company to approach us was Bharat Biotech. The Bharat Biotech proposal was an exciting one as it fitted well with the Indian government's publicly stated prioritization of indigenous technology, production and capabilities in all sectors. I personally knew Krishna Ella, founder and chairman of Bharat Biotech, as a competent scientist, a good researcher who had returned from the US in 1996 and set up this model biotech firm in India. We had a common friend from Stanford University, where he worked on the Rotavirus vaccine project. I had been engaged with the bio-design programme with Stanford University with certain mentors there, to develop low-cost medical devices and we were successful in developing several such devices through a fruitful collaboration of engineers and doctors. Thus, we were familiar with each other's work culture. This medium-sized private vaccine maker based in Hyderabad proposed to join hands with the ICMR to produce a COVID-19 vaccine. Bharat Biotech already had a track record of producing a range of vaccines for neglected diseases such as rotavirus and typhoid. Thus, Bharat Biotech had the experience and it was the only manufacturing facility in the country which had a BSL-3 laboratory and BSL-3 is the basic prerequisite for building a killed virus vaccine for COVID-19.

'There was an environment that was charged with possibilities, for this collaboration. The time was demanding and the environment was ready,' Dr Samiran Panda recalls.

THE IDEAL PARTNER

Bharat Biotech International Ltd (BBIL) is the brainchild of its chairman, Dr Krishna Ella. Dr Ella is a molecular biologist who returned to India in 1996 after working as a researcher in the US, where he had conceptualized a new hepatitis B vaccine.

Bharat Biotech's first major success was to produce the hepatitis B vaccine[3] at prices affordable to low-income countries in Asia and Africa.

The company, based in Hyderabad, was launched with just ₹12.5 crore as its seed capital. Within three years, its first hepatitis vaccine was out in the market. Sold at ₹10 per dose to India's national immunization programme, the vaccine was one of many the company would develop and launch in the following years. Today, Bharat Biotech has over 700 employees, comprising research scientists and manufacturing professionals. It owns 160 global patents, exports to over 65 countries and has delivered more than three billion vaccine doses all over the world.

'Our company's mission is to deliver affordable, safe and high-quality vaccines and bio-therapeutics that help people prevail over diseases,' Dr Krishna Ella proudly said.

The company's next major vaccine was Rotavac, to protect against the highly contagious rotavirus, which causes infant diarrhoea in many low-income countries. The vaccine was the product of a unique joint venture between Indian and international researchers as well as public and private sectors and sold at just $1 per dose.

'I believe that partnering between public research institutions and private companies is essential to produce good science as they can help validate each other,' says Dr Krishna Ella. According to him, Rotavac demonstrated that an Indian company could conduct high-quality research in advanced sciences.

Subsequently, Bharat Biotech also went on to produce a low-cost vaccine for typhoid, a neglected tropical disease. The company was among the first to initiate developing vaccines for viral diseases like chikungunya and Zika. Today, besides Covaxin, the company is involved with three other COVID-19 vaccine development initiatives.

WHY AN INACTIVATED VIRUS VACCINE?

We wanted Bharat Biotech to work on an inactivated virus vaccine. It turned out to be the perfect choice.

Inactivated vaccines are developed by 'killing' the lab-grown, well-characterized virus using chemicals and subsequently generating a product with a known concentration of inactivated viral particles. These destroy the pathogen's ability to replicate, but keep it 'intact' so that our immune system can still recognize it and produce an immune response. These inactivated viruses are then reproduced in large quantities and prepared for use as a vaccine.

'We have produced almost 500 million doses of inactivated virus vaccines for rabies, Japanese encephalitis, rotavirus and polio over the years. So, we have plenty of experience working with this technology,' Dr Krishna Ella informed.

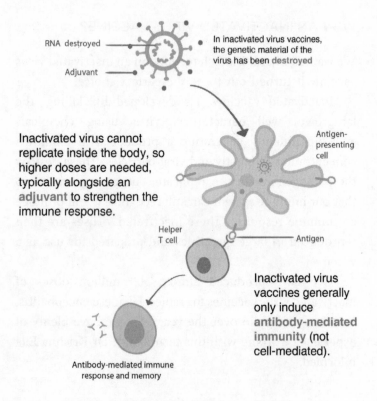

RNA destroyed

Adjuvant

In inactivated virus vaccines, the genetic material of the virus has been destroyed

Inactivated virus cannot replicate inside the body, so higher doses are needed, typically alongside an adjuvant to strengthen the immune response.

Antigen-presenting cell

Helper T cell

Antigen

Inactivated virus vaccines generally only induce antibody-mediated immunity (not cell-mediated).

Antibody-mediated immune response and memory

Figure 6.1: How inactivated virus vaccines work

IT'S SAFE ...

The ICMR and Bharat Biotech's decision to go for a vaccine using an inactivated virus was based on other considerations as well. Inactivated vaccines are among the earliest vaccines developed, starting in the late nineteenth century. They have been licensed for decades with well-established safety profiles as they don't contain any live components. You won't get any nasty surprises and there is no chance of getting the disease from the vaccine. They can be given to special populations such as infants, pregnant women and the geriatric population.

Making an inactivated virus vaccine does take a lot more time than the new messenger RNA or mRNA technology used by several global vaccine makers. Preparing large quantities is more challenging as manufacturers have to cultivate large batches of the virus before inactivating them.

... AND ROBUST TOO!

The whole inactivated virus used in the vaccine was also expected to have a greater chance of dealing with mutant varieties of the SARS-CoV-2 virus. As the virus evolves, the spike proteins on its surface can also change, a big concern when we consider the efficacy of vaccines aimed solely at neutralizing the spike proteins.

One advantage of the inactivated virus-based vaccines such as Covaxin is that they stimulate antibodies that target not just the spike proteins of SARS-CoV-2 but also other features on the virus's surface. This makes them more likely to be effective even if the virus and the spike protein undergo mutations over time, though this theory is yet to be confirmed through further studies. We have however demonstrated the efficacy of this vaccine against the notorious variants: alpha, beta, gamma and delta.

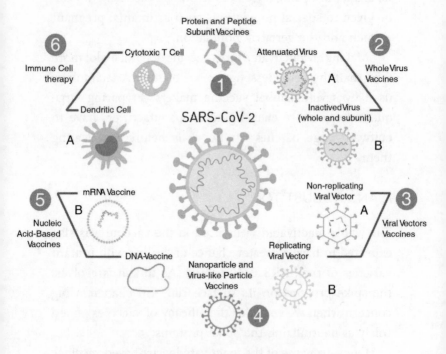

Figure 6.2: Platforms for developing COVID-19 vaccines

GLOBAL VACCINE INITIATIVES

Many researchers all over the world are working on COVID-19 vaccines. The global vaccine pipeline for COVID-19 has more than 112 vaccine candidates in clinical trials and 185 in preclinical development.[4] This includes live attenuated, killed, subunit protein, mRNA and recombinant vaccines.

Some of the most prominent vaccines from this long list include those produced by companies such as Moderna, Pfizer, Astra Zeneca and Johnson & Johnson, all of which use very different platforms.

The Moderna and Pfizer vaccines use mRNA technology, considered a promising alternative to conventional vaccine approaches because of their high potency, capacity for rapid development and potential for low-cost manufacture and safe administration.[5]

The Oxford-AstraZeneca vaccine places the gene segment responsible for producing the coronavirus spike protein inside a modified, inactivated version of a chimpanzee adenovirus that can enter human cells, but can't replicate inside them.

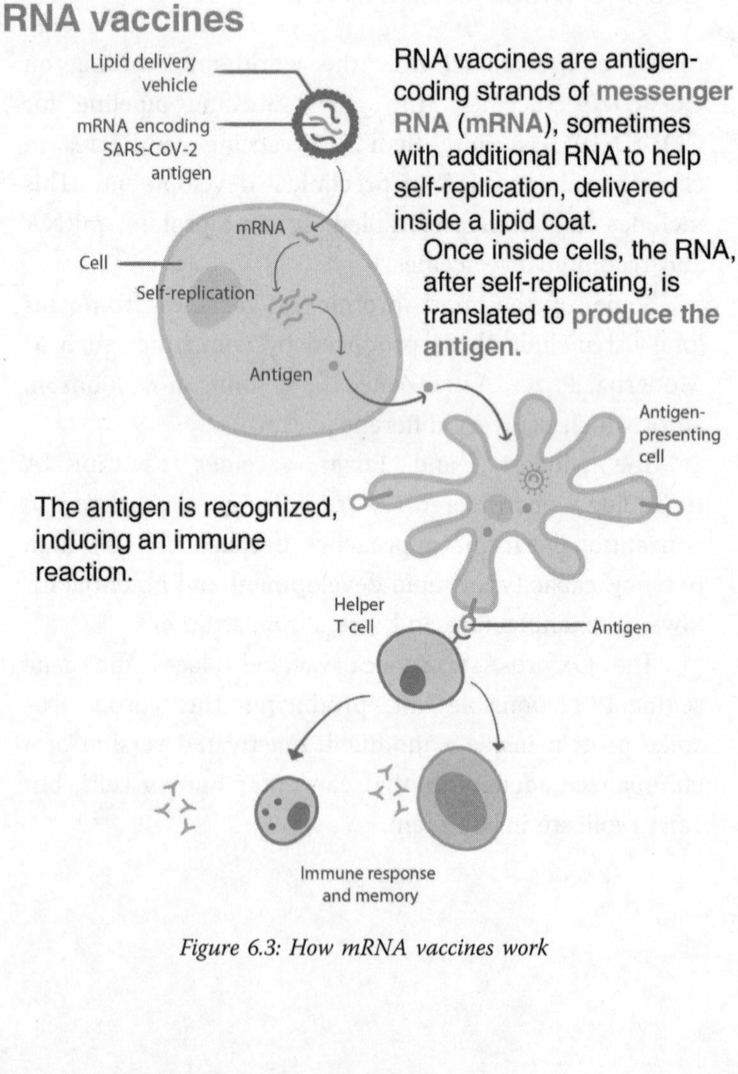

RNA vaccines

Lipid delivery vehicle

mRNA encoding SARS-CoV-2 antigen

mRNA

Cell

Self-replication

Antigen

RNA vaccines are antigen-coding strands of messenger RNA (mRNA), sometimes with additional RNA to help self-replication, delivered inside a lipid coat.

Once inside cells, the RNA, after self-replicating, is translated to produce the antigen.

Antigen-presenting cell

The antigen is recognized, inducing an immune reaction.

Helper T cell

Antigen

Immune response and memory

Figure 6.3: How mRNA vaccines work

Unlike the other vaccines, including Covaxin, which are administered in two doses several weeks apart, the Johnson & Johnson vaccine is effective with just a single shot.

It was a conscious decision not to rely on Moderna, Pfizer or Johnson & Johnson because, first of all, they were limited in their production. Second, those vaccines required a very high cold chain of minus 70 degrees Celsius, which was a problem as far as India's infrastructure was concerned. Covaxin can be stored at normal refrigerator temperatures. Scientists are also looking at vaccines which could be stored at room temperature.

Developing a vaccine for COVID-19 on our own was also hugely attractive as it would reduce both import costs and dependency on overseas suppliers or governments. While India was already known as the 'pharmacy of the world' for its export of low-cost generic medicines and vaccines, it did not have many entirely home-grown products. This was an opportunity to show to the world India's ability to come up with a cutting-edge product developed with exclusively domestic expertise and resources. We wanted to save lives. We also wanted to do our country proud. Despite all the constraints, a few things worked in our favour. As luck would have it, Bharat Biotech had set up a high-quality manufacturing platform in Hyderabad to make injectable polio vaccines just before the COVID-19 pandemic struck. The company had also set up a BSL-3 laboratory for virus propagation at minimum risk. Its personnel quickly repurposed those facilities to help with the indigenous vaccine project.

The ICMR–Bharat Biotech partnership was destined to be an iconic Indian success story: a fruitful arranged marriage! The company had collaborated with the ICMR several years earlier for the development of JENVAC—an inactivated virus vaccine for Japanese encephalitis.

Bharat Biotech had the track record of making vaccines. Thus, we decided to share the virus with the firm and characterize the company's vaccine by partnering with the Indian company. An MoU was put in place regarding the sharing of intellectual property (IP) rights. It was decided that five per cent of the earnings from the sales would be given to the ICMR. I think it was one of the first agreements of its kind where both the IP rights and the sales earnings were shared in the manufacture of a vaccine.

We constantly updated the agreement, for instance when we supplied to Bharat Biotech the variants—whether it be the Delta or the Delta plus variant—so that they could tweak the vaccine accordingly to meet the challenge of the new variants.

FIRST TESTING STEP: SMALL ANIMALS

Once the BBIL-ICMR-NIV team developed three inactivated SARS-CoV-2 vaccine candidates (BBV152A, BBV152B and BBV152C), it tested them on small animals like mice and rabbits. The goal was to see if the test animals produced neutralizing antibodies that provided any protection when subsequently challenged with the live virus.

BBV152B induced significantly high concentrations of neutralizing antibodies in all animal models tested, without any safety issues.[6] The vaccine was evaluated at three antigen concentrations, and including two adjuvants. Then, it was tested on Syrian hamsters;[7] it was chosen for study as the SARS-CoV-2 virus replicates well in both its upper and lower respiratory tracts.

The hamsters produced significant amounts of antibodies that neutralized the SARS-CoV-2 virus.[8] The vaccine clearly provided protection to the hamster, by rapidly clearing the virus from the lower respiratory tract and reducing virus load in the upper respiratory tract. The vaccinated animals' lungs were undamaged. Out of the three candidates, BBV152A was the winner.

Strict quality control ensured that nothing went wrong at any point of time. Anti-SARS-CoV-2 ELISA test kits developed by ICMR-NIV were used for preclinical studies that required detecting antibodies generated following vaccination.

From ICMR headquarters, we kept a regular watch on the entire process. We monitored the work and sprang into action to expedite the necessary approvals and ensure supplies of critical equipment and materials, including reagents.

SERIOUS MONKEY BUSINESS

It is important to remember that this story's heroes are not just human ones. Twenty monkeys are partly responsible for the fact that millions of us now have access to a life-saving vaccine.

Once we knew that the vaccine could generate antibodies in small animals, the next logical step was to test it out on larger animals such as monkeys, comparable to humans in terms of their body structure and immune systems. The data from these studies would help supplement what we would learn from human trials about the vaccine's safety and efficacy. If the data was good, we could speed up the process of getting the vaccines out of the lab and into people's upper arms.

The Rhesus macaque monkeys, used worldwide in medical research, were the best non-human primates for such studies. The ICMR-NIV's BSL-4 lab, the only state-of-the-art facility in India for primate studies, once again took up the challenge to carry out this critical research. While it looks simple on paper, experimenting on monkeys is a

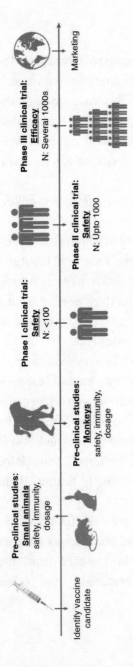

Pre-clinical studies: Small animals
safety, immunity, dosage

Pre-clinical studies: Monkeys
safety, immunity, dosage

Phase I clinical trial: Safety
N: <100

Phase II clinical trial: Safety
N: Upto 1000

Phase III clinical trial: Efficacy
N: Several 1000s

Identify vaccine candidate

Marketing

- Normal vaccine development occurs in 4-5 years
- Fast-tracking of various steps in pandemic
- EUA, combine phases, parallel studies, use of established platforms

Figure 6.4: How the vaccine development process works

complex endeavour. First, researchers have to consider the ethical implications and decide whether they can justify carrying out the experiments. In this case, though the choice was clear to the scientists, they still had to deal with multiple objections raised by animal rights groups. They also had to navigate plenty of red tape, which was facilitated by the government.

What wasn't so clear was: where to get the monkeys from?[9]

India does not have laboratory-bred Rhesus macaques. NIV researchers contacted multiple zoos and institutes all over India to find some. They didn't have any luck. Just to make things more difficult, they needed young monkeys with a good immune response, as a couple of ageing monkeys at the NIV were unsuitable.

A dedicated team from ICMR-NIV travelled to areas of Maharashtra to identify sites for animal capture. Macaques, losing their usual urban food sources because of the lockdown, had gone deep into the forests. The Maharashtra forest department helped to track them down, scanning several square kilometres of forests for days to track the monkeys, before finally finding them near Nagpur.

Protecting the experimental animals from SARS-CoV-2 before starting the preclinical studies was another challenge. As the animals could be infected from the humans, all the caretakers, veterinarians and other cleaning staff were screened for SARS-CoV-2 weekly, and had to follow strict prevention protocols.

Performing large animal experiments in the NIV's high-security containment facility was the next challenge. To begin with, this required developing critical infrastructure (bronchoscope, X-ray machine, appropriate housing for monkeys), training the team, developing protocols, standardizing procedures like bronchoscopy in macaques and performing the necropsy.

There were a lot of balls in the air and we couldn't afford to drop any. We had to plan very carefully. It was exhausting as well as tough to perform these experiments in the positive pressure suits, in the containment facility for 10–12 hours without food and water. NIV also did not have the in-house expertise to perform some of the studies required. They asked for and got help from doctors at the Armed Forces Medical College in Pune.

In the end, everything fell into place. The monkey business was accomplished, and the participants of both species who made it possible deserve more praise than we could possibly give them.

Twenty Rhesus macaques were divided into four groups of five each. One group was administered a placebo—which did not have any active substance meant to affect their health—while three groups were immunized with the three different BBV152 vaccine candidates at 0 and 14 days. All the macaques were exposed to SARS-CoV-2

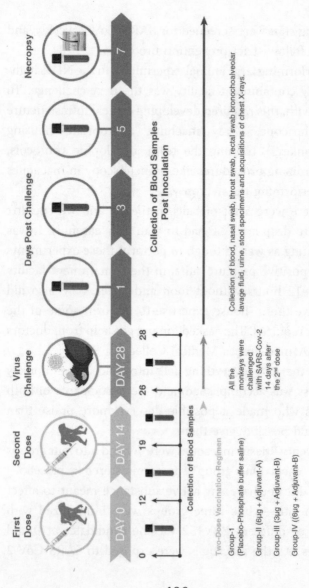

Figure 6.5: Testing the vaccine on non-human primates

14 days after the second dose. The virus was delivered deep into the lungs via bronchoscope.

The macaques had strong immune responses to the vaccine. They were protected when they were exposed to the virus. The vaccinated primates cleared the virus well from their lungs, nasal and throat passages within seven days of being infected.[10] Daily bronchoscopy with lavage was taken from deep in the lungs.

The vaccinated groups, unlike subjects in the placebo group, did not develop pneumonia. Overall, the vaccines showed remarkable immunogenicity and protective efficacy. It was a turning point for all of us at the ICMR and Bharat Biotech. It was one of the best results that we had encountered. The vaccinated monkeys showed excellent antibody response with no adverse effect.[8] We thereafter concluded that the vaccine was both safe and effective, and that with the new adjuvant it could be administered in the dose of either three or six micrograms.

We finally had a completely indigenous vaccine, an epitome of *Atmanirbhar Bharat*.

7
THE MOMENT OF TRUTH

Once the small animal studies were successful, Bharat Biotech moved quickly with the Drugs Controller General of India (DCGI) to carry out human trials using the most promising vaccine candidate. In June 2020, the company got permission to conduct Phase I and Phase II human trials, 12 sites were selected for randomized, double-blind and placebo-controlled clinical trials of the potential vaccine.

Clinical development of vaccines is a three-phase process:

Phase I: Small groups of people receive the trial vaccine. These are trials to determine the safety of the vaccine. Such trials can be undertaken with more than one vaccine formulation.

Phase II: A few hundred people are vaccinated, to understand the immune response triggered by the vaccine formulations. Safety is also, once again, studied simultaneously. The winning formulation goes to Phase III trials.

Phase III: Thousands of people get the vaccine, testing for efficacy as well as safety and immunogenicity.

Many vaccines also undergo yet another phase, Phase IV post-marketing surveillance studies, after the vaccine is approved and licensed.

755 individuals participated in the Covaxin Phase I and Phase II clinical trials, which began in July 2020. For the trials, due to safety and ethical concerns, we only included healthy individuals. We followed all the ethical principles for biomedical research that involves human participation. We did not involve anyone from the vulnerable population, such as children, pregnant mothers or any other vulnerable groups. All individuals who participated in the trials came voluntarily.

Both trials reported that the vaccine candidate BBV152 worked well. The vaccine induced binding and neutralizing antibody responses. We were thrilled that the prestigious international peer-reviewed journal, *The Lancet Infectious Diseases*,[1] [2] published our results, including the added bonus that the adjuvant in the vaccine worked exactly as we had hoped on the human immune system. Now we were sure: the vaccine was safe and efficacious.

UNDERSTANDING VACCINE IMPACT

The three Es of vaccine benefits are efficacy, effectiveness and efficiency.

Efficacy refers to the vaccine's working under ideal conditions, i.e., in the laboratory or other clinical settings. Typically, a vaccine is tested on a group of consenting participants who are enrolled in the efficacy trial following pre-determined inclusion and exclusion criteria. A control group that does not receive the intervention serves as a comparison group.

Effectiveness addresses how the vaccine works when administered in a real-world setting. This is because, although under controlled conditions efficacy may be satisfactory, (as described above) a real-life setting could produce different results. This may be due to the fact that people did not complete the course of the vaccine as prescribed or due to the administration of the vaccine in diverse population groups, whereas the efficacy trial may have been conducted in a more or less homogeneous population.

While the vaccine may be shown to be effective, is it possible to achieve the intended treatment outcomes in a cheaper or better way? Efficiency addresses the costs of the new vaccine versus its benefits. At the same time, it is important that the vaccine triggers the desired immunity.

The human body has two kinds of immunity: natural (innate) and acquired (adaptive).

If you think of the body as a fortress, prepared against an army of viruses or other toxins, then the natural immune system provides the first line of defence against invaders. The most capable soldiers of the natural immune system include leukocytes (white blood cells), dendritic cells, natural killer cells and plasma proteins.

They can detect viruses and bacteria as soon as those invaders enter the body.

The natural immune system also plays a key role in triggering a response from the acquired immune system with either chemical signals called cytokines, or parts of infectious organisms called antigens.

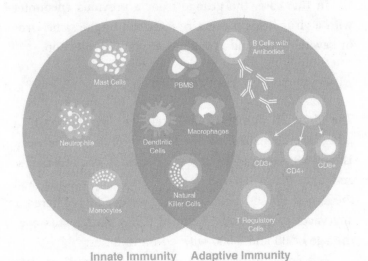

Innate Immunity   Adaptive Immunity

Figure 7.1: How the human immune system works

These provoke the acquired immune system to produce antibodies, which are basically Y-shaped proteins, released by our body's cells into blood and mucosa. They bind like a lock-and-key to the microorganisms and disable or destroy them.[3] Different antibodies are produced for battling different pathogens in very targeted ways.[4]

The adaptive immune system builds a memory bank of cells for easier recognition and attack in the event of future exposure. T and B cells do this work. These cells, like us, have memories, and, also like us, can hold a grudge.

In this case, the grudge from a previous encounter with a virus helps prevent re-infection by the same virus or severe illness and provides long-term protection.

ALMOST THERE: PHASE III TRIAL

The Phase III human clinical trials of Covaxin began in mid-November 2020, involving 26,000 volunteers, between 18 and 98 years of age, across 21 sites. It was India's first and only Phase III study for a COVID-19 vaccine, and the largest Phase III efficacy trial ever conducted here for any vaccine. The study included 2,433 participants over the age of 60 and 4,500 with co-morbidities.

The interim results of the trial released[5] in late April 2021, showed an efficacy of 100 per cent against severe COVID-19 disease; the efficacy of protection from asymptomatic COVID-19 infection was 78 per cent, putting it at par with other global front-runner vaccines. The analysis was on a data set of 127 Covid-positive volunteers.

Data from 25,800 participants, half of whom received

the vaccine and the other half a placebo, also showed that the vaccinated candidate was safe and well tolerated. A review of the safety database showed that severe, serious and medically attended adverse events occurred at low levels and were balanced between vaccine and placebo groups. This was again published in *The Lancet*.

Analysis from the NIV indicated that vaccine-induced antibodies could neutralize the known variants of concern including the delta variant.[6]

This was all excellent news! Those results will always be a matter of great pride to us at the ICMR, which I will cherish for the rest of my life. There were critics who said that we had to complete Phase III before giving the vaccine to humans, before it could be given to the nation. But there is a Gazette notification of 19 March 2019, which is pre-COVID, and it said that in national interest, if a product has successfully undergone the Phase II trial, it can be deployed. In other words, emergency authorization can be given. And that rule was invoked by the Drugs Controller on 2 January 2020, when approval for Covaxin was issued.

The leadership had about, I would say, more than 15 meetings with various chief ministers of different states. And at that point in time, we had to participate and any question that was put forward for the vaccine or for the testing would come to me. So we were all on our toes at every level. But there was no question after the Emergency

Use Authorization (EUA) happened. We were only asked how we could help out; the government would help the company to scale it up.

As we battled one challenge after another and found ways to deal with them, and firmed our resolve to have an Indian vaccine, a tiny section of our population—the so-called experts in the media and elsewhere—began to raise doubts on our ability. It was not the first time that an Indian initiative was being ridiculed even before it had the opportunity to succeed. But it was disgraceful that it should happen at a time when our scientists and researchers were showing a steely determination to find a solution to the pandemic.

It was the Macaulay-mindset at work. What had T.B. Macaulay done? He framed India's education policy. He said that if the East India Company had to rule over this country, we have to systematically destroy its education system, drilling every Indian's mind that the Indian education system is inferior to that of the British. This was instilled in 1834 in every Indian's mind. It is this Macaulay mindset which is responsible for every Indian critic in India who feels that anything Indian can never work.

And that's why I told Bharat Biotech in a lighter vein, that they should name their company after 'another country' Biotech not Bharat, for acceptability from the Macaulay-minded people! It was something I mentioned during my depositions before the Department Related Parliamentary Standing Committee on Health and Family Welfare and the parliamentary standing committee on 'COVID-19 pandemic response, India's contribution and the way forward'. I would like to put on record that the members of these panels were most supportive and praised the efforts of the ICMR. Cutting across party lines, they were also of the opinion that the work that the ICMR had done was phenomenal.

Once the Phase III clinical results came out, it laid to rest the criticism of the cynics. It is the vaccine which has more than 10 full scientific publications in top international journals, all featuring only Indian authors.

The approvals for Covaxin, contrary to criticism, were purely data-driven. Phase II trials established beyond doubt the immunogenicity of the vaccine. No responsible Subject Expert Committee (SEC) approves vaccines without adequate data, and those involved with the approval were all responsible people. Experts had taken into account the alpha variant of SARS-Cov-2 before granting approval to Covaxin. And because Covaxin is a whole-virus inactivated vaccine, as I mentioned earlier, it is equipped to target all parts of the virus instead of just partially. The virus is known to have undergone mutations in the spike protein also, and drug makers such as Pfizer Inc. have admitted that it needs about four to six weeks to make tweaks to their vaccine to adjust to the new mutations.

MAKING THE VACCINE

Bharat Biotech's long experience in developing and manufacturing inactivated virus vaccines enabled it to dive confidently into the Covaxin project.

'We already had three licensed vaccines based on this technology, including an oral rotavirus vaccine, supplied in huge volumes to the Government of India. We also exported to Africa and South America,' said Dr Raches Ella, head of Business Development and Advocacy at Bharat Biotech. The other two were vaccines for Japanese encephalitis and rabies.

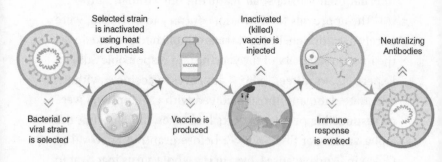

Figure 7.2: The inactivated virus vaccine production process

The manufacturing process consists of culturing the virus in large quantities in a Vero cell platform, inactivating the virus chemically, and then filtering the resultant solution to get the vaccine, which is essentially the inactivated virus combined with appropriate adjuvant. It is the ultimate healthy cooking: a pinch of this, a spot of that and stir the pot.

Bharat Biotech's state-of-the-art manufacturing facility in Genome Valley, Hyderabad, is the largest facility of its kind in the Asia-Pacific region. It is no exaggeration to say that it is a factory for magic potions.

Safety and efficacy are both paramount. The first goal is to make sure the infectious virus is completely inactivated. This is done by repeatedly testing batches of inactivated viruses in the lab.

Second, technicians must make sure that they conserve the important parts of the virus, relevant for provoking a good response from the human immune system. This is critical to get an antigen, which will result in the production of the required type and quantity of antibodies as well as stimulate cell mediated immune response after receiving the vaccine. In other words, a delicate balance has to be maintained between the immune system's response and preventing the vaccine itself from causing severe illness of any kind.

One of Bharat Biotech's innovations to the conventional inactivated virus production process had to do with pharmacological agents called adjuvants, which are added to vaccines to boost the immune response. Aluminium hydroxide or alum is generally the adjuvant of choice for many inactivated vaccines, but these can lead to undesirable inflammatory response caused by Type 2 T-helper cells or TH2.

To avoid this problem, Dr Ella suggested incorporation of a novel adjuvant in the vaccine. Sunil David, researcher and founder of biotechnology company ViroVax had developed the new adjuvant called Algel-IMDG. This particular adjuvant has been shown to enhance vaccine efficacy without leading to undesirable immune responses, but had never been used in any vaccine before.[7]

There was no literature on the subject. We tested it at different doses—three micrograms, six micrograms, etc. All permutations and combinations were tried out.

We took the calculated gamble of using that adjuvant in our new vaccine for the first time in the world. The Chinese vaccine is identical to the Indian vaccine in terms of the whole virus, but it doesn't have this novel adjuvant. With this formulation of the BBV152 vaccine, the team found both higher levels of virus-neutralizing antibodies and good T-cell responses, promising long-term protection for those who take the vaccine.

Several experts and editorials in the media across the world praised the innovation.[8] This adjuvant featured as a cover story in the reputed science journal *iScience*.

VIRUS-NEUTRALIZING ANTIBODIES

During the clinical trials, NIV provided critical technical support by testing serum samples from vaccinated people for neutralizing antibodies, an important defence against viral invaders in the human immune system.

Neutralizing antibodies are among those few that bind to a virus in a way that effectively blocks infection.[9] Following an infection, it usually takes some time for the host to produce highly effective neutralizing antibodies, but these stay for a long period and provide protection against future infection from the virus.

'Measuring the concentration of such neutralizing antibodies that can block virus replication is an important way of understanding the extent of protection provided by vaccines,' Dr Gajanan Sapkal, senior scientist at NIV Pune said. The plaque reduction neutralization test, which utilizes the ability of a specific antibody to neutralize a virus, is considered the gold standard for detecting and measuring neutralizing antibodies.

In this test, different dilutions of the human sera sample are mixed with a constant amount of virus and placed on top of a layer of Vero cells. While normally the virus forms a plaque on the layer, in this case it can't do so wherever the antibodies manage to neutralize the virus. The percentage of plaques formed to the overall estimate of virus used tells us how effective the antibodies are.

While this entire endeavour was a grim race against time with very high stakes, it was also an unforgettable professional experience for many of the people involved—from government offices to private institutions. The Covaxin story is also a story of human compassion and cooperation.

India has a long history of academia-industry collaboration in the field of pharmaceutical research and production, but in vaccine development this trend has been relatively sparse. The different work cultures of private and public institutions can be a big barrier to their working together.

However, the ICMR's experience of working with BBIL was extremely wonderful with total transparency in all our communications and interactions. Many of my senior colleagues have characterized the collaboration with BBIL as 'one of the strongest public-private partnerships that the ICMR ever experienced' and marked by 'trust, transparency and timeliness'.

The admiration is reciprocated fully by Dr Krishna Ella, who says he is very impressed by the professionalism of the scientists working with ICMR-NIV.

'The people we worked with at NIV were proactive and not only capable but very quick with the work they did, and speed was really essential in our project for the new vaccine,' says Dr Ella.

Our communications with BBIL were really on a daily

basis, to review our progress along with ideation for further action. We also had regular meetings with the directors of our research institutes to ensure the timely performance of the sero-surveys as well as the clinical trials.

My major point of contact at Bharat Biotech was their managing director, Dr V. Krishna Mohan, a brilliant scientist trained at Cambridge. I would talk with him in detail everyday at 10.00 a.m. We would discuss the developments and the roadmap ahead, all of that I managed, while also being engaged in writing manuscripts, approving the manuscripts, the publications, the clinical trials and the funding. It was hard but satisfying work.

We would talk with Dr Ella once in 15 days, or once in a month to sort out issues related to problems that the firm had with the government, or other matters. We were always there to help. Dr Ella later said that several steps in the vaccine development process simply could not have happened without the help of the ICMR scientists.

For example, soon after the NIV handed over the stock of the new virus, Bharat Biotech evaluated the genetic stability and adaptability of the SARS-CoV-2 strains to grow in higher concentrations. Next, the virus was inactivated and purified, and the BBIL technical staff prepared different vaccine candidate formulations.

The NIV researchers then examined these vaccine candidates for their various properties using neutralizing antibody assays, through electron microscopy and other laboratory studies. These results, together with various protocols, assays and reagents were shared with counterparts at Bharat Biotech.

ICMR-NIV also carried out the preclinical studies in animal models such as hamsters and Rhesus macaques. Apart from providing the special facilities required ICMR was also responsible for obtaining various ethical clearances for these studies.

More recently, in early 2021, ICMR-NIV scientists isolated the new mutant varieties of the SARS-CoV-2 that have been detected in the UK[10] and Brazil, and which could have implications for the efficacy of all the vaccines cleared for public use. While studies so far show the efficacy of Covaxin holds up well against most of these mutant viruses, both BBIL and ICMR-NIV staff continue to monitor and update findings.

EFFICACY AGAINST NEW VARIANTS

All RNA viruses, including SARS-CoV-2, mutate or change over time. Most changes have little to no impact on the virus' properties. However, some mutations may affect the way the virus behaves, such as how easily it spreads, the associated disease severity, or the performance of vaccines, therapeutic medicines, diagnostic tools.[11] WHO has labelled virus strains carrying such mutations, as variants of concern (VoCs) in order to prioritize global monitoring, research and inform the ongoing response to the COVID-19 pandemic.

The bulk of the cases recently recorded in different parts of India as part of the second wave of COVID-19[12] are believed to be due to highly transmissible B.1.617.2 variant, called 'delta' in the WHO's new naming system.[13] The WHO has described delta variant as a VoC. Besides the delta variant, other VoCs include the alpha variant,[14] first detected in the UK; beta variant, detected initially in South Africa and gamma variant detected first in Brazil.

In order to assess the protective efficacy of Covaxin against the VoCs, the ICMR-NIV undertook a study to evaluate the neutralization potential of antibodies in blood samples of Covaxin vaccinated individuals against the live variant virus culture samples.

The researchers measured the levels of neutralizing antibodies in the vaccines against the original SARS-CoV-2 strain and compared the neutralizing potential of these antibodies against the four VoCs. Findings of the study demonstrated that the neutralization potential of Covaxin against the alpha VoC was at par with the original SARS-CoV-2 strain. The results further suggested that as compared to the original strain, the neutralizing potential of Covaxin was reduced against beta, gamma and delta VoCs, but still the antibody titres were good enough to neutralize these VoCs.

'The COVID-19 vaccines have set the record for fastest

development of any vaccine in history,' Dr Krishna Ella said, with a justifiable amount of pride. He pointed out that in normal times it would take close to 10 years to develop a vaccine, sequentially carry out all the different trials required for safety and efficacy and then get the necessary regulatory clearances.

However, the pandemic created an urgent need for expedited approaches worldwide. Innovative designs were instituted by researchers and industry wherein established and previously tested platforms of vaccine development such as prequalified cell lines, vector backbones, recombinant gene approaches, virus like particles, nanoparticles, lipid envelopes and tested adjuvants were used. Additionally, preclinical and clinical development pathways were run concurrently and not sequentially, cutting down the timeline to about 10 months.

The Indian regulator, DCGI, adopted the innovative mechanism of a 'rolling review' of data emerging from ongoing vaccine trials, to speed up the process of authorizing new vaccines for public use. It also devised strategies for granting EUA on humanitarian grounds in a public health emergency, while prioritizing science and ethics.

For example, the DCGI accorded EUA to two vaccines, Covishield and Covaxin, on the first two days of 2021, following which India became one of the global leads in COVID-19 vaccine introduction. The rules safeguarding the integrity and ethics[15] of medical research are the toughest among regulatory mechanisms anywhere.[16] This is simply because anything to do with medicine is usually a matter of life and death and only the highest standards are acceptable.

However, in the kind of dire health crisis created by the COVID-19 pandemic, such rules worldwide have had to be tweaked to speed up research or clinical trials that may be of great public benefit if proven successful.[17] This calls for innovations to regulatory processes that may never have been tried out earlier under normal circumstances, with uncompromised scientific quality, participant safety and ethical practices.

For example, in the course of the COVID-19 pandemic, several therapies that showed promising results were approved by Indian drug regulators under the EUA powers vested with them. This was done on the grounds that the known and potential benefits of the therapy outweighed its known and potential risks. However, some of these were also withdrawn subsequently with availability of new research that showed their benefits were not significant enough.

An innovation to the rules was similarly required, when the developers of Covaxin presented their implementation plan, after completion of animal studies to check for safety and efficacy, to test out the vaccine on human subjects. The clearance was given[18] in early 2021 under the novel concept of 'clinical trial mode', used for the first time in India. This was done while the Phase III trials of the vaccine were ongoing and clinical efficacy was yet to be established.

While giving it the green light, the Central Drugs Standard Control Organization (CDSCO), which approves all new drugs and clinical trials in the country, imposed various restrictions and conditions to be followed. It stipulated, for example, that the vaccine be used after informed consent of the individual and all recipients be followed for safety and tracking of adverse events.

Since the term 'Clinical Trial Mode', was used for the first time by the CDSCO, there were still many grey areas regarding its meaning, components and implementation. To help obtain greater clarity the ICMR-Central Ethics Committee on Human Research (CECHR) decided to put together a panel of experts to discuss its implications, especially concerns regarding medical ethics and also the implementation modalities.

Recommendations from the experts focused on measures to minimize risk and improve transparency and accountability. These included a simple yet fully informative consent form—translated into all Indian regional languages—and distribution of good quality advocacy and information material for better public understanding of the trial process.

8

RISE OF A VACCINE SUPERPOWER

ndia's emergence as one of the world's biggest vaccine producers is built on a long history of the country's involvement with research and development related to many important vaccines since the late nineteenth century. Even before that, vaccination was a part of our heritage—we were performing variolation, a crude precursor of vaccination, thousands of years ago![1]

For example, the world's first effective vaccine with few severe side effects for cholera was tested and established in India between 1893 and 1896 by Dr Waldemar Haffkine, a bacteriologist who had developed it while studying at the Pasteur Institute in Paris.

Dr Haffkine vaccinated more than 40,000 people in Calcutta (now Kolkata) as part of his clinical trials, and the vaccine was accepted by the medical community. Dr Haffkine also went on to discover the world's first plague vaccine in 1897.[2]

By the late nineteenth century, apart from the existing plague vaccine research unit at the Grant Medical College in Mumbai set up by Dr Haffkine, the smallpox vaccine lymph was being produced in Shillong (since 1890), now the capital city of the northeastern state of Meghalaya. In 1899, the King Institute of Preventive Medicine and Research in Chennai also established facilities for production of vaccines against various infectious diseases. In the early twentieth century, at least four vaccines—for smallpox, cholera, plague and typhoid—were available in the country.

In view of the growing vaccine requirements, the colonial Indian government decided to set up new vaccine institutes. In 1905, the Central Research Institute was set up in Kasauli, Himachal Pradesh, followed by the Pasteur Institute of Southern India in Coonoor in 1907.

Legend has it that the death of a young English woman, Lily Pakenham Walsh, who died of hydrophobia in the year 1902, because she could not get anti-rabies treatment in time, led to the establishment of the Pasteur Institute. American philanthropist Henry Phipps donated ₹50 lakh to Viceroy Lord Curzon for the development of medical institutions.[3] One lakh of this was allocated to start the Pasteur Institute in southern India.

While initially focusing solely on production of the anti-rabies vaccine, the Pasteur Institute went on to develop and manufacture influenza vaccines and trivalent oral polio vaccines. It also conducted landmark research in the production of tissue culture and then Vero cell-derived DNA purified rabies vaccine for human use. Since 1977, the institute has functioned as an autonomous body under the MoHFW, Government of India.

Soon after Independence, tuberculosis was perceived

as a major cause of morbidity and mortality in the country. As a response, in 1948, it was decided to set up a BCG Vaccine Laboratory at the King Institute in Chennai to introduce BCG vaccination on a limited scale. Over the decades, the institute played a major role in the battle against tuberculosis throughout India. Even today, it manufactures Freeze Dried BCG vaccine for the control of childhood tuberculosis and tuberculous meningitis.

The network of government-supported institutes made India a global pioneer in vaccine development and ensured both self-reliance and low-cost vaccine production. The range of vaccines produced included those against diphtheria, polio, tetanus, typhoid, smallpox, cholera, tuberculosis, Japanese encephalitis and yellow fever, among other diseases. New vaccines under development include those meant to combat dengue, Zika and chikungunya.

Even in the very early days of the Covid pandemic, when everything was unknown, experts were sure about one thing: with regard to vaccines, India would surely play a key role in their mass production and distribution to the rest of the world.

This is not entirely surprising, given the steadily growing profile of India as the 'pharmacy of the world'. Over the last several decades, the country's pharmaceutical industry has emerged as the third largest in the world in terms of medicines produced by volume, and fourteenth by value. We have an established domestic pharmaceutical industry, with a network of 3,000 drug companies and more than 10,500 manufacturing units.[4] The domestic pharmaceuticals market turnover reached US$20.03 billion in 2019[5] and India also contributed the second-largest share of the world's pharmaceutical and biotech workforce. India is also the world's largest provider of generic drugs, and as of late 2020, the country exported pharmaceuticals worth almost US$11 billion, 20 per cent of the global generic drug exports, most of it to North America.[6] However, it is in the production of vaccines that India's global domination is astounding, accounting for over 60 per cent of the global demand[7] and supplying high quality but low-cost vaccines to more than 150 countries around the world.

Although we are the pharmacy of the world, in most cases we are mainly generic product makers. We are not making new molecules. We are the pharmacy of the world because we are able to make expensive products, less expensive. And we are able to give them to the rest of the world, for example, we supplied the HIV drugs to all of Africa. With Covaxin, we proved that we could manufacture vaccines from start to finish, with the virus that has been isolated by an Indian scientist. The virus was isolated in an Indian lab and the vaccine was manufactured in an Indian lab. It was characterized in an Indian lab by an Indian scientist. It was studied in India on small and then large animals. The Phase I, II and III clinical trials were done in India by Indian scientists. Almost all the ingredients were from India, as far as the vaccine was concerned.

Covaxin is a hardcore, purely-homegrown product. In today's inter-connected world, you can source the globe for certain components. But to be able to innovate, to be able to own the Investigational Product (IP) and to be able to manufacture it on your own, that is a feat, and we did that with Covaxin. Look at the journey and one will understand the stellar achievement:

THE JOURNEY

March 2020: SARS-CoV-2 virus is isolated by scientists at ICMR-NIV, Pune. India becomes the fifth country in the world to achieve this feat.

April 2020: ICMR-NIV Pune signs an agreement with BBIL, for the development of whole-virus inactivated vaccine for COVID-19.

May 2020: ICMR-NIV transfers the virus strain to BBIL and characterizes the vaccine developed by BBIL through in-vitro experiments and electron microscopy studies.

June 2020: Covaxin is the first coronavirus vaccine created in India to be approved for clinical trials.

June–August 2020: Experiments in small animals (mice, rats and rabbits) and hamsters established safety and immunogenicity of Covaxin.

July 2020: A Phase I and II clinical trial begins with 755 participants.

September 2020: Results from studies in Rhesus macaques establishes safety and protective efficacy of Covaxin.

October 2020: The Company announces a Phase III trial with up to 26,000 participants.

November 2020: Phase III clinical trials are initiated.

December 2020: Covaxin's Phase I and III trials show the vaccine produces antibodies to the coronavirus without causing serious side effects.

January 2021: The Indian government grants Covaxin emergency authorization, in keeping with international guidelines.

16 January 2021: India rolls out phase-wise COVID-19 vaccine administration starting with healthcare and frontline workers.

27 January 2021: Covaxin's ability to neutralize UK variant strain of SARS-CoV-2 is established.

3 March 2021: Interim results of Phase III efficacy trials of COVAXIN show 81 per cent efficacy against SARS-CoV-2 virus. The follow-up of participants in the trial is ongoing.

Looking back, the quest to becoming a vaccine superpower was fuelled by the Prime Minister's faith in the country's scientific community. He would repeatedly say that he would only and always go by scientific decisions—whether it is scaling up testing, rapid antigen tests or restrictions.

THE PRIVATE SECTOR BOOM

Apart from Bharat Biotech, currently seven other Indian vaccine makers are involved in major vaccine production ventures. 'While there are many countries producing vaccines, only India has the capacity to produce sufficient quantities to satisfy the demands of citizens globally,' Dr Krishna Ella observed.

Consider the HIV epidemic. India, by mass-producing affordable generic antiretroviral drugs, made 'an extraordinary contribution to human well-being,' noted Stephen Lewis, former United Nations Special Envoy for HIV/AIDS in Africa, adding, 'With Covaxin, once again, India emerges as a potential saviour.' While historically, it was the public sector that led the way, in the last couple of decades many new players from the private sector have also ventured into vaccine production in a big way. Bharat Biotech is a good example of this phenomenon.

Indian companies can produce vaccines much cheaper than their competitors abroad, and they have become the biggest suppliers of essential vaccines procured by large international organizations such as the Global Alliance for Vaccines and Immunization (GAVI) and the United Nations Children Emergency Fund (UNICEF).

The UNICEF's procurement of vaccines from India has grown at a compound annual growth rate (CAGR) of 25.3 per cent between 2003 and 2014. Other global agencies have also upped their orders as much over the same time.

'Our research, manufacturing and clinical trial costs are much lower than what large pharmaceutical companies in developed countries incur, and this enables us to sell large volumes,' a senior researcher at a large Indian vaccine production company said.

Active assistance from various government bodies also helps Indian vaccine makers keep their costs low. Currently, the Indian government supports vaccine research and development initiatives through government funding agencies like our own ICMR, the Department of Biotechnology (DBT) and the Indian Council of Agricultural Research (ICAR).

Spurred by the prospect of global sales, Indian firms have also strengthened their capabilities in biotechnology, built collaborations with international partners and moved from basic vaccines to more sophisticated technologies. Currently, more than two-thirds of the total volume of the vaccines manufactured in India is exported, while the rest is used domestically.

WORLD'S LARGEST VACCINATION PROGRAMME

India's roll-out of COVID-19 vaccines has been the largest adult vaccination program in the world—an almost indescribably complex and massive undertaking.

While Indian academia and industry were working to develop high-quality vaccines, the Indian government set up a system to make it real—to make and deliver inoculations up and down the subcontinent, from snowy villages to sun-soaked fishing hamlets.

A National Expert Group on Vaccine Administration for COVID-19 (NEGVAC) was set up by the NITI Aayog along with the MoHFW to address several key issues. These included vaccine delivery, selection, procurement, prioritization, cold chain logistics, finance and equity, both domestically and globally.

The committee was established in August 2020 to deliberate on various issues related to vaccines. What vaccines should be important? What vaccines should be manufactured? What should be scaled up? Which should be approved? What should be the guidance for approval? What should be the export policy? What should be the import policy? These and several other queries were to be addressed by the NEGVAC committee headed by the health secretary and member NITI Aayog and chairman, National Task Force Prof. (Dr) V.K. Paul.

Additionally, public health officials were trained. A

web-based vaccine delivery management system, called CoWIN, with user registration, reporting and tracking of adverse events and certificate generation, was introduced.

And all this happened while we were working tirelessly to get the vaccine to those who needed it most urgently. Thirty million healthcare and frontline workers and 270 million people over 50 years old were prioritized[8] for vaccine delivery in the Phase 1 roll out plan, which was launched in mid-January 2021. Since 1 May 2021, access to vaccines was extended to all those over 18 years of age and on 21 June 2021, the Government of India also announced that all adults over the age of 18 will be vaccinated for free.

For me, it was a very emotional moment while taking the vaccine. My eyes filled up with joy. It was a proud moment for every Indian, but at that point in time, we didn't have the Phase III results. So, there was a sense of apprehension too. I was not worried about the side effects. I was more worried about the efficacy being established, because with Covaxin being a killed virus vaccine, I knew that there were not going to be side effects or deaths due to the vaccine. I told my people that, whatever work they did, they must publish it and file it, so that it is peer reviewed and the world believes in it. That is exactly what happened with us. We have 10 papers on Covaxin, and we have another four or five papers on the variants, which are now part of the world literature and will be there for posterity.

The day the Prime Minister took Covaxin, was indeed a happy day for me. When vaccination was opened up for his age group, after the health workers and frontline workers, he took the vaccine. At that time, we did not have the Phase III results. His action addressed the scepticism of a lot of critics.

My wife would tell me, if India had not manufactured the vaccine, we would be going around the world seeking help and who knows what would have been the situation in the absence of a vaccine. We are lucky that we have our own home-grown vaccine that is saving the lives of millions.

If you look at the COVAX (a worldwide initiative aimed at equitable access to COVID-19 vaccines directed by Gavi, the Vaccine Alliance (formerly the Global Alliance for Vaccines and Immunization, or GAVI), the Coalition for Epidemic Preparedness Innovations (CEPI), and the World Health Organization (WHO) data, those that are taking vaccines from different parts of the world— January, February, March, April data—70 per cent of the vaccines are from India. Our supply to the world stands at 28 per cent of the vaccine; just one per cent has been from the UK and the US. For most, charity begins at home, but we also supplied to the world as we catered to the domestic requirement. This was our vaccine diplomacy. This was done when there was initial vaccine hesitancy and we had a large stockpile.

If we had not manufactured a vaccine, just imagine the situation: 1.4 billion people and no vaccines available. We would have been going around, pleading with the US, the UK and others to give us vaccine. They would have put their own interests first. Would China have given us vaccines? And even if they had given, it would be at steep prices.

Those were emotional moments. The slogan used by the top leadership at Indian Science Congress, *Jai Jawan, Jai Kisan, Jai Vigyan, Jai Anusandhaan* (Hail the Soldier, Hail the Farmer, Hail the Science, Hail the Research) inspired the whole effort which signifies the importance of research.

COMMUNICATING DURING THE PANDEMIC

'If you can't explain it simply,
you don't understand it well enough.'

—Albert Einstein

Taking a cue from the quote, the ICMR rapidly made strides to enhance its capacity in health communications. However, I did not anticipate the magnitude and relevance of communications, especially when I had joined the organization. Whenever a health issue occurred in any part of the country, a beeline of reporters would ask us questions. Though our role was primarily research—health management and implementation in synergy with the national programs and COVID-19 was no different. But considering the importance of health communication to create awareness among the masses ICMR had already initiated the Health Communication Ecosystem within the organization and a Communication Unit was already set up in the Headquarters in 2016 linked with all the ICMR Institutes with Nodal Communication Officers (NCOs) helping in communication related activities, that proved as a boon during the pandemic situation as many of our scientists were trained in communication through this initiative.

We were busy with the work and along with that we planned our communication strategy so as to keep the media and the public updated on the day-to-day activities. As an immediate response, we created a new dedicated webpage for COVID-19 where all the information related to COVID-19, including advisories and guidelines were made available.

Questions from the media, including international media and TV channels were replied on top priority, press briefings/press releases were issued as and when needed. Communication through social media was also accelerated. All the ICMR institutes remained connected with Headquarters and we were having virtual meetings to understand the needs of the institutes and what needs to be communicated to the society. Op-eds and popular articles in newspapers and popular magazines were also brought out from time to time. We became active on Twitter as well.

We were all in uncharted waters: a global pandemic, a national public health emergency. I cannot even recall a health crisis in the past, where scientists were the face of responding to queries about health emergencies. COVID-19 could easily be the first one for India, where scientists doubled up as communicators—the ICMR became a household name.[9]

The ICMR learned from the past and was open to communications as and when we could. The problem with scientific communications is a bit more complex. However, there were few challenges as well, unless we have the results of a trial or a research study, we can't really communicate what the results could like—if we do this it would be scientifically blasphemous, but we also didn't want people to accuse us of withholding information. This constant dilemma was the story of communicating in the pandemic.

For example, the Indian health authorities' decision to provide EUA to Covaxin, before complete data on efficacy from its Phase III trial was available, was based on an assessment of public health benefits of such a move. This was also done according to 'New Drugs and Clinical Trials Rules 2019'—it states that during a public health emergency, a drug or vaccine could be approved for emergency use on the basis of Phase II trials. These rules came out much before the COVID-19 pandemic stuck the country. However, the authorization was construed as being an attempt to push a 'dodgy' product and bordering on the 'unethical', when similar authorizations have been given to newly developed vaccines all over the world.

The fact remains that we pulled off something fantastic—an indigenous vaccine, safe and effective. Many richer nations did not even try this, preferring to throw money around to try and corner as much of the vaccine market as they could from a handful of private pharma companies. Poorer nations face an inordinately long wait before they can get to vaccinate their citizens.

One of the consequences of the public and often unfounded doubts about the quality, efficacy and safety of Covaxin, has been some reluctance to get vaccinated. Though the criticism of the EUA was not the only factor involved, it lent weight to existing vaccine hesitancy due to ignorance, misinformation and unfounded fears. In fact, we have proven beyond doubt that the vaccine is safe. A sore arm and a day's worth of fever is the worst that could happen, and I would venture that most people would prefer that than death by COVID. Or worse, being responsible for a loved one's death due to COVID.

Dr Samiran Panda writes, 'there cannot be a one-size-fits-all approach to vaccine hesitancy.'[10] He notes that this is not a new phenomenon, and that a key element is the building of public trust through clear and transparent communication, and great attention to correct messaging. This involves empathy rather than judgement, and positive rather than negative inducements. The ICMR played a critical role in communicating the benefits of vaccination[11] and, in turn, tackling hesitancy. We worked with the MoHFW and produced evidence-based collaterals and communication programmes like *Vaccine Varta*. In this dynamic and ever-evolving pandemic, we ensured only scientifically proved messaging went out to the public.

Following the release of the interim Covaxin efficacy data, and as suspicions about its safety melt away, it is only a matter of time before public confidence in the vaccine grows strong. The ICMR and other Indian research institutions have learned a valuable lesson: it is not enough to do good science. We also need mastery over the subtle (and sometimes not so subtle) art of communication.

DEALING WITH THE 'INFODEMIC'

The nationwide lockdown was announced on 23 March 2020 by the government of India. There was suspicion, tension and curiosity as nothing much was known about the disease called COVID-19. As the pandemic progressed, queries started pouring in from regional media houses across India. Besides the scientists and general public, the

Indian media too naturally had a lot of questions.

There was concern about the testing—whether we had sufficient reagent and kits, enough stock of primers and probe, whether non-vegetarian food should be stopped, about the protocol for wearing masks and social distancing, etc. Other questions were regarding international travel, testing of patients with respiratory illness, contact tracing, availability of labs, reinfection, quality of testing kits, migration of workers, the containment zone strategy and vaccine development.

The flood of media queries was the most in the initial days of the national lockdown. There was too much confusion and too many questions; high-speed answers were needed with evidence and sound scientific basis.

'Calls came even at odd hours, late at night, enquiring about the latest update, seeking clarity or sound bites from the ICMR Director General and other scientists,' recalled Dr Rajni Kant, head of communications at ICMR.

The ICMR communication team improvised its response, providing round-the-clock information through direct contacts as well as social media messaging, press release and by creating a separate webpage for COVID-19 information on the ICMR website.

This proactive approach helped immensely in tackling the 'infodemic' that has characterized the COVID-19 pandemic in many parts of the world, due to misleading information, fake news and rumours. Later, the ICMR launched a special newsletter in English and Hindi, named *E-Samvad* that published the latest research updates. Regular virtual meetings with the ICMR nodal communications officers and other scientists further improved media communication at the regional as well as national level.

'We made sure that updated information reached the public without creating a scare,' Dr Kant said.

LOOKING AHEAD

The ICMR has had a storied 111-year history. It is one of the oldest institutions of its kind anywhere in the world, with a long list of achievements to its credit. It was founded in 1911 as the Indian Research Fund Association, and renamed in 1949. The central role played by the ICMR and its various units in helping tackle the crisis have made us household names in India today.

'Innovative health solutions identified through research conducted by the ICMR, since its inception, have helped in changing the landscape of public health in India in numerous ways and in areas of both communicable and non-communicable diseases,' says Dr Samiran Panda.

In 1947, India faced a variety of challenges on the health front, many of them related to poverty and lack of basic infrastructure at a time of low food production and rapid population growth. Over the years, through a visionary political leadership, the dedication of thousands of health personnel and the participation of ordinary citizens, India has come a long way in dealing with these crises.

Even in those early days, scientists at the ICMR working on problems of malnutrition, infectious diseases and health policy played a quiet and unassuming role in the background. Over the years, its researchers have carried out valuable work in a wide variety of disciplines from virology and epidemiology to drug efficacy and disease prevention, adding to global medical knowledge in significant ways.

From oral rehydration therapy for diarrhoea to short-course chemotherapy for TB, research done by the ICMR scientists' stands out as work that has had worldwide impact. Often working in tandem with global collaborators, ICMR researchers have helped tackle a diverse range of health threats from tuberculosis, malaria, kala-azar and leprosy, to pandemics like HIV, the highly pathogenic Nipah virus disease and now the COVID-19 pandemic.

The ICMR believes that our researchers must understand the pressing needs and gaps in various public health programmmes and conduct research in tandem with policy makers. Often the critical questions for which the policy makers require immediate answers are not addressed by researchers. There has been a huge communication gap, with the two groups working in silos.

During COVID-19, we bridged some of these gaps by synthesizing evidence to inform intervention development such as use of face mask[12], reopening of schools[13] or responsible travel versus 'revenge travel'[14]. These made rounds in local regional and national print media as well as social media platforms and facilitated public engagement in debates and discussion around finding the way forward.

While all this takes experience, it also needs passion and a new vision. As Dr Samiran Panda puts it, 'While these examples underline the immense capacity of India in conducting quality research, there is always room for improvement. One area that specifically comes to my mind is encouraging a research-oriented curriculum at the school and college level'.

In this vein, the ICMR is keenly aware of the importance of young scientists and wants its Institutes to open up and enable young and competent people to exercise their minds and think freely. It is only with such freedom that young scientists will be inspired to make meaningful contributions to public health. We have some of the world's smartest young people here. Let's do everything we can to help them live up to their amazing potential. That will be the great initiative in the seventy-fifth year of India's Independence.

HIGH QUALITY AT LOW COST

As in the past, India's innovations in the health and pharmaceutical sectors reverberate around the globe for a very simple reason—they lower the costs of access to quality healthcare for some of the poorest people anywhere in the world.

At the ICMR, one of our primary goals is to make the price of medicine and medical devices in India the global benchmark, so that it is possible for everyone in the world, irrespective of income status, to access modern healthcare. ICMR scientists are focusing on developing high quality and effective but inexpensive drugs, implementing digital health solutions and a variety of assistive technologies.

Looking into the future, we envisage India as a global leader in innovation and production of frugal technologies, i.e., low-cost solutions for common diseases affecting large groups of people. And the way to achieve this lofty goal is by focusing on doing good quality research on a host of diseases that are endemic to countries of the Global South, but neglected by richer nations as part of their 'not my problem' syndrome.

SPINOFFS FROM THE COVID EXPERIENCE

In the quest to develop an indigenous vaccine, the ICMR embarked upon an innovative path. Some of the studies that we carried out were completely new to our teams. For example, the testing of candidate COVID-19 vaccines on non-human primates and the follow-up investigations were new experiences for the NIV researchers. During 2020, apart from the animal facility within its BSL-4 laboratory, the institute was upgraded with state-of-the-art medical, surgical and essential laboratory equipment to undertake new studies.

I am certain that the rapid acquisition of skills and infrastructure will also benefit the country in tackling future pandemics.

Epilogue
THE REAR-VIEW MIRROR

On 10 December 2020, I tested positive and was admitted to the trauma centre of the All India Institute of Medical Sciences. I had fever, and so the doctors wanted to admit me. An ambulance came to pick me up. Sadly, there was no one who could accompany me. I took a small bag and went to the trauma centre. It was freezing cold. Though all the doctors and nurses were good and kind, I was all alone for about seven days in the hospital, communicating with my wife and children over the phone.

I realized the trauma of being totally alone with a disease, and attached with it a stigma. I was so weak that getting back to work soon seemed impossible.

Today, more than nine months later, the COVID-19 saga is still not over. We know this all too well, having lived through India's terrible second wave, where we all lost loved ones and colleagues.

We have to stay alert. We have to keep doing intensive research. We continue to monitor the new SARS-CoV-2 strains. We continue to detect resurgences. We continue to test, test and test again. We continue to identify COVID-19 hotspots and institute timely containment measures. We carefully follow vaccination patterns to learn more about how it works.

I have detailed the journey, examined and analysed the process, and laid out the groundwork for the future.

We pulled off an extraordinary feat. After the tension, the drama, the hard work, the long nights, the constant fear of illness and death, the brainstorming, the travel, the testing, the fatigue, the adrenalin rush... after all this, let's pause and marvel. There is much to marvel at.

Last year, we had one lab that could perform COVID-19 tests. Today, we have several thousands.

Last year, a deadly disease came to our country and started killing people, and it was a terrifying mystery. Today, we know exactly what the 'pretty virus' is and exactly how to vanquish it. The lives lost, and the lives still in the balance are an incalculable loss, but now we know what to do.

Last year, the whole world shut down. This year, India has an Indian vaccine that will save millions of lives all over the globe and help the world come back to life.

Last year, we were known as a reliable vaccine manufacturer. This year, we are an acknowledged vaccine pioneer.

Today, I am filled with a sense of urgency to vaccinate India and prevent a repeat of the tragic second wave. We have to be very careful.

Ironically, the best way forward for us is to imitate our enemy: we need to mutate and evolve in order to outsmart the virus. And that is what we are doing. When it attacks, we defend. When it hides, we find it. When it changes course, we are right there behind it. When we need to, we call in reinforcements.

At this moment, as the world waits to see the pandemic in the rear-view mirror, the superheroes of the day are scientists: women and men who stay smarter than the virus, who change and adapt and innovate so we can all have our shot at a better tomorrow.

ACKNOWLEDGEMENTS

This book would not have been possible without the tremendous work done by the institutes under the aegis of the Indian Council of Medical Research (ICMR).

While weaving this story, I received valuable inputs, information, interesting anecdotes and suggestions from many colleagues at the ICMR as well as at Bharat Biotech International Ltd (BBIL). Among those I would like to mention from the ICMR are Dr Samiran Panda, Dr Nivedita Gupta, Dr Priya Abraham, Dr Rajni Kant, Dr Pragya Yadav, Dr Gajanan Sapkal, Dr Varsha Potdar, Dr Gururaj Deshpande and Dr Enna Dogra Gupta. In BBIL, my special thanks go to Dr Krishna Ella and Dr Raches Ella for agreeing to be interviewed and providing their viewpoint. Mirza Shadan and Sohini Pal and Sanya Sodhi from Global Health Strategies (GHS) played an important role in shaping the book and helping in illustrations.

I am immensely grateful to Satyanarayana Sivaraman and Sohaila Abdulali for helping me prepare the draft of the book and offering bright ideas in between the chapters as well as in collecting information through phone/video calls. I also acknowledge Pradeep Kakkatil of the Joint United Nations Programme on HIV/AIDS (UNAIDS), Dr Swarup Sarkar, ex-C G Pandit Chair, ICMR and Ex-Director, WHO-SEARO and Kaushik Bose, Global Health Strategies (GHS) for facilitating the financial support in engaging them for this project. I thank Simran Tapadia for providing support in the preparation of graphics.

I would also like to thank my peers and colleagues in institutions with which the ICMR has always worked closely, such as the Central Drugs Standard Control Organization and the Ministry of Health and Family Welfare.

I would like to express my sincere thanks and gratitude to all the participants who were enrolled in this vaccine's trials as well as the Institutions involved, which made it possible to see light at the end of the long tunnel.

Last but not the least, I am indebted to my family who stood like a pillar and provided untiring support to me during the testing times.

NOTES

PROLOGUE: TAKING THE BULL BY THE HORNS

1. Andrews, MA, et al., 'First Confirmed Case of COVID-19 Infection in India: A Case Report', *Indian Journal of Medical Research*; Vol. 151, No. 5, 2020, pp. 490–492.
2. 'Daily COVID-19 Tests', *Our World in Data*, https://ourworldindata.org/grapher/full-list-covid-19-tests-per-day.
3. Madhaikar, Manisha et al., 'India's Crusade Against COVID-19' *Nature Immunology*, Vol. 22 No. 3, March 2021, pp. 258–259.
4. 'Pneumonia of Unknown Cause—China', WHO Disease Outbreak News, 5 January 2020, https://www.who.int/emergencies/disease-outbreak-news/item/2020-DON229.
5. Yadav, Pragya D, et al., 'Full-genome Sequences of the First Two SARS-CoV-2 Viruses from India', Indian Journal of Medical Research, Vol. 151, No. 2, April 2020, pp. 200–209.
6. Gupta, Nivedita, et al., 'Strategic Planning to Augment the Testing Capacity for COVID-19 in India', *Indian Journal*

of Medical Research. Vol. 151, No. 2 & 3, February 2020, pp. 210–215.

7. Gupta, Nivedita et al., 'Laboratory Preparedness for SARS-CoV-2 Testing in India: Harnessing a Network of Virus Research & Diagnostic Laboratories', Indian Journal of Medical Research, Vol. 151, No. 2 & 3, March 2020, pp. 556–565.

8. 'Reported Cases and Deaths by Country, Territory, or Conveyance', As of 3 January 2021, *Worldometer*. https://www.worldometers.info/coronavirus/?.

9. 'Mortality in the Most Affected Countries', Coronavirus Resource Center, Johns Hopkins University of Medicine, https://coronavirus.jhu.edu/data/mortality. Accessed on 3 January 2021.

10. 'Reported Cases and Deaths by Country, Territory, or Conveyance', *Worldometer*, https://www.worldometers.info/coronavirus/?. Accessed on 25 January 2021.

1: PREPARING FOR THE APOCALYPSE

1. 'Pneumonia of Unknown Cause—China', WHO Disease Outbreak News, 5 January 2020, https://www.who.int/emergencies/disease-outbreak-news/item/2020-DON229.

2. Jain, Vijay Kuma, et al. 'Differential Mortality in COVID-19 Patients from India and Western Countries', *Diabetology & Metabolic Syndrome*, Vol. 14, No. 5, September–October 2020, pp. 1037–1041. DOI: 10.1016/j.dsx.2020.06.067.

3. Pathak, Sanmoy et al. 'Countries with High Deaths Due to Flu and Tuberculosis Demonstrate Lower COVID-19

Mortality: Roles of Vaccinations', *Human Vaccines & Immunotherapeutics*, Vol. 17, No. 9, September 2021, pp. 2851–2862. DOI: 10.1080/21645515.2021.1908058.

4. Brooks, Nathan A., et al. 'The Association of Coronavirus Disease-19 Mortality and Prior Bacille Calmette-Guerin Vaccination: A Robust Ecological Analysis Using Unsupervised Machine Learning', *Scientific Reports*, Vol. 11, January 2021, https://doi.org/10.1038/s41598-020-80787-z.

2: CORONAVIRUS: THE SCIENCE EXPLAINED

1. Racaniello, Vincent. 'The Abundant and Diverse Viruses of the Seas', *Virology Blog*, 20 March 2009, https://www.virology.ws/2009/03/20/the-abundant-and-diverse-viruses-of-the-seas/.

2. Jones, Kate E. 'Global Trends in Emerging Infectious Diseases. Nature, 451, February 2008, pp. 990–93. DOI: 10.1038/nature06536.

3. 'Prioritizing Diseases for Research and Development in Emergency Contexts', https://www.who.int/activities/prioritizing-diseases-for-research-and-development-in-emergency-contexts.

4. Waleed, M. Sweileh, 'Global Research Trends of World Health Organization's Top Eight Emerging Pathogens', *Global Health*, Vol. 13, No. 1, February 2017. DOI: 10.1186/s12992-017-0233-9.

5. Sadanadan, Rajiv et al., 'Towards Global Health Security: Response to the May 2018 Nipah Virus Outbreak Linked to Pteropus Bats in Kerala, India', *BMJ Global Health*, Vol. 3,

No. 6, November 2018. DOI: 10.1136/bmjgh-2018-001086.

6. Mourya, Devendra T. et al., 'Emerging/Re-emerging Viral Diseases & New Viruses on the Indian Horizon', *Indian Journal of Medical Research*, Vol. 149, No. 4, April 2019, pp. 447–467.

7. Thangaraj, Jeromie W.V. et al., 'A Cluster of SARS-Cov-2 Infection among Italian Tourists Visiting India, March 2020', *Indian Journal of Medical Research*, Vol. 151, No. 5, May 2020, pp. 438–443.

8. Sarkale, Prasad et al., 'First Isolation of SARS-Cov-2 from Clinical Samples in India', *Indian Journal of Medical Research*, Vol. 151, No. 2 & 3, February–March 2020, pp. 244–250, https://www.ncbi.nlm.nih.gov/pmc/articles/PMC7366528/.

9. Dr Pragya Yadav from ICMR-NIV, Pune remembers,

> As soon as cytopathic effects (visual signs of virus growing) were observed in 11 samples, the tissue culture fluid was tested for SARS-CoV-2 and confirmed by real-time RT-PCR. Prasad Sarkale, Srikant Baadkar, Rajen Lakra and I stood in front of the machine to see if the cyclic threshold amplification plot would go high. Once it showed CT of 10, Prasad cried out in delight. We had a small tea party later.
>
> The team could not sleep with excitement as it was about to open a big research avenue for creating reagents of ELISA, pathology study, antiviral test development and, most importantly, vaccine development. But the main confirmation by

sequencing was still pending and those two days were spent in total suspense. As soon as genome data and phylogenetic analysis was analysed, a message was immediately sent to Dr Priya Abraham, director, and Prof. Balram Bhargava on the achievement. Growth kinetics, virus titration and morphological analysis by electron microscopy were performed within a few weeks. The virus was used to raise immune serum in mouse and rabbit animal's models.

10. Prasad, Sharda et al., 'Transmission Electron Microscopy Imaging of SARS-Cov-2', *Indian Journal of Medical Research*, Vol. 151, No.2 & 3, February–March 2020 pp. 241–243.

11. Pišlar, Anja et al., 'The Role Of Cysteine Peptidases in Coronavirus Cell Entry and Replication: The Therapeutic Potential of Cathepsin Inhibitors', Vol. 16, No. 11, November 2020, https://doi.org/10.1371/journal.ppat.1009013.

12. Hamming, I et al., 'Tissue Distribution of ACE2 Protein, the Functional Receptor for SARS Coronavirus. A First Step in Understanding SARS Pathogenesis', *The Journal of Pathology*; Vol. 203, No. 2, June 2004, pp. 631–637. DOI: 10.4103/ijmr.IJMR_577_20.

13. Sapkal, Gajanan et al., 'Development of Indigenous IgG ELISA for the Detection of Anti-SARS-Cov-2 IgG', *Indian Journal of Medical Research*, Vol. 151, No.5, pp. 444–449. DOI: 10.4103/ijmr.IJMR_2232_20;

14. Dr Pragya Yadav from ICMR-NIV, Pune remembers,

Dr Anita Shete, Dr Rajlaxmi Jain and their teams worked tirelessly to develop ELISA for the screening of mouse, hamster and the Macaque serum for the testing of IgM and IgG antibody. In the meantime Dr Gajanan Sapkal's team members were provided refresher training to work in BSL-3 facility of Maximum Containment Facility. We provided them the virus and the support and they came out with PRNT50 and MNT assay, which become a handy tool for vaccine study.

15. Murhekar, Manoj V. et al., 'Prevalence of SARS-Cov-2 Infection in India: Findings from the National Serosurvey', *Indian Journal of Medical Research*, Vol. 152, No. 1 & 2, May–June 2020, pp. 48–60. DOI: 10.4103/ijmr.IJMR_3290_20;
16. Dr Srikant Kanungo from ICMR-RMRC, Bhubaneswar recounts his experience,

As part of the fourth National sero-survey by the ICMR, our centre was assigned three districts in Odisha. When one of our team reached a place called Jirudia in Rayagada district, along with the local healthcare workers, they were welcomed with verbal abuses from the residents, who were totally ignorant about the concept of surveillance. They simply said that they won't give their blood samples and that we were preparing to cart them away to the hospitals. Some people just shut their doors, while others ran away towards a mountain near the village. The team had to wait for four hours without any collection.

A media person captured the views of children

and people from the village running towards the hill. The reason for their non-cooperation was the stigma associated with the pandemic. Gradually, after thorough counselling and motivating for two to three hours, people started to cooperate and we finally returned home after achieving the target.

17. Murhekar, Manoj V. et al., 'SARS-Cov-2 Antibody Seroprevalence in India, August–September, 2020: Findings from the Second Nationwide Household Serosurvey', *The Lancet Global Health*, Vol. 9, No. 3, March 2021, 257–266, https://doi.org/10.1016/S2214-109X(20)30544-1.

18. Murhekar, Manoj V. et al., 'SARS-Cov-2 Sero-Prevalence among General Population and Healthcare Workers in India, December 2020–January 2021', International Journal of Infectious Disease July 2021, pp. 145–155.

3: TESTING TIMES

1. 'How India Scaled Up Its Laboratory Testing Capacity for COVID19', World Health Organization News, 16 August 2020, https://www.who.int/india/news/feature-stories/detail/how-india-scaled-up-its-laboratory-testing-capacity-for-covid19.

2. Dr Anup Anvikar from ICMR-NIMR, New Delhi recalls his experience,

Covid had entered India in the last week of January 2020. I was asked to hunt for Viral Transport Medium (VTM) for about 400 quarantined persons arriving from China. As days passed, everyone was worried about contracting the SARS-CoV-2 infection and the consequences thereof. The situation in many countries was scary. I used to sit right inside the fever clinic, where we also used to receive international travellers as patients.

I was asked to establish COVID-19 testing laboratory at my institute (ICMR-National Institute of Malaria Research). Cases were being reported from more and more states. A nationwide lockdown was eminent. There was a surge in demand for basic equipment for COVID-19 lab, as these items were required by many players for establishing facilities for testing. There was a shortage of supplies in the market. It was difficult to even get masks, let alone PPE and other lab supplies. If they were available, they were overpriced. Despite the challenges, we succeeded in establishing the lab in March, 2020.

Simultaneously, I was entrusted with establishing a COVID-19 reagents depot at my institute, which was later on converted into a Central Depot. We used to get large consignments of various kits, and had to send smaller ones to different parts of the country. We used to closely work with Customs officials, logistic personnel and airlines. There used to be special flights operated for carrying the kits to places. I do remember sending our vehicles to other states with the kits. It was a proud feeling to facilitate testing at various labs situated even in distant places like Andaman and Nicobar Islands, Ladakh and northeastern states.

On one evening in March, I received a letter from the ICMR headquarters, asking me to report with immediate effect to the National Institute of Biologicals, Noida, for coordinating the Covid testing and reporting. It was 40 kilometres from my house. Throughout my service, I stayed on the campus or in the vicinity of the office. I thought this was a different kind of work, and would be challenging. It was a great opportunity to utilize my expertise in managing the pandemic.

Reporting was the biggest challenge, as all the stakeholders wanted the reports at the earliest. Many times, the last rites of the deceased would be pending due to the non-availability of the Covid report. Timely reports were required for patient care and to prevent further spread. I got a good team from the NIMR as well as the NIB, making the operations smoother. Further, I got to know the NIB better.

There were no weekends, public holidays, leave or vacation for more than a year. There were times when I would not go home for three to four days at a stretch. My wife had to visit hospitals or community centres for Covid-related activities. Due to the lockdown, there was no household help; children were unable to attend school. It was quite a challenge to manage work and home in such a situation. We mentally prepared our children and said they might have to stay alone at home or in quarantine facility, if any of us got infected.

During lockdown 1.0, very few vehicles/people used to leave their residential society for work. People used to be curious about me and ask: 'You go to hospitals and labs. You have to deal with samples from patients. Are you not scared?' Of course, we were scared. But those were also days when I was really proud to be a doctor, and an ICMRian. No one was allowed on the roads, but by the virtue of being doctor, my vehicle used to get access anywhere. The ICMR became a household name. My senior colleagues used to give press briefings. Many more people came to know that I worked for the ICMR, and they admired me for that.

Later, it was enjoyable to work on different aspects of COVID-19 management: collecting the specimens for testing, visiting different hospitals for specimen collection, establishing the Biorepository, training the health staff in carrying out antigen tests and also assessing them, coordinating testing in community, coordinating research projects and so on.

During the 20 years of my career in malaria research, I have been hearing about a possible malaria vaccine. It takes a long time for a new vaccine to hit the market. However, COVID-19 vaccines have been developed really fast—and this is especially true of the indigenous Covaxin. When vaccines were being developed abroad, we were happy but also unsure about their availability in India. The cost also bothered us. What about the ultra-low temperatures required for their storage and transport? We heard talks of some manufacturing to happen in India. This way, we could have got some doses available in India. Then came the breakthrough. An Indian vaccine, Covaxin, a totally made-in-India product, was in the pipeline. I really felt proud to be an ICMRian.

3. 'Charité/Berlin (WHO) Protocol Primer and Probe Panel', Integrated DNA Technologies, https://eu.idtdna.com/pages/landing/coronavirus-research-reagents/who-assays.

4. Choudhary, Manohar L. et al., 'Development of In Vitro Transcribed RNA as Positive Control for Laboratory Diagnosis of SARS-Cov-2 in India', *Indian Journal of Medical Research*, Vol. 151, No. 2, April 2020, pp. 251–254.

5. Dr Kamran Zaman from ICMR-RMRC, Gorakhpur looks back on and shares his story,

Beep (WhatsApp msg in COVID-19 lab group): 'Number of samples received 3,500, and total sample labelled/opened by evening receiving team 2,200'. What a pleasant alert message to get on a late evening! It was the result of joint efforts and hard work for almost more than a year, ever since we started testing in March 2020.

The story started back on the New Year Eve of

2020, when the world encountered the SARS-COV2 infection in Wuhan, China; which was later named COVID-19. India reported its first case in January 2020. This was when our laboratory received a request for testing samples of two China-returned Indian students in the Maharajganj district. The samples were sent to NIV Pune as there was no lab in all of Uttar Pradesh for testing COVID-19.

With increasing cases of COVID-19, the ICMR led the country from the front, by establishing more COVID-19 testing laboratories. RMRC Gorakhpur, a regional research institute of the ICMR in eastern UP, was given the responsibility to establish a COVID-19 lab. Since we had no well-equipped BSL-2 plus lab facility in our institute, we collaborated with the microbiology department of BRD Medical College to set up a lab, utilizing the college's BSL-2 plus facility.

Following training and validation of the control results, we started testing on 23 March 2020. On the first day, we received five samples, followed by one sample the next day. Receiving samples itself was a tale. I used to get a call from the chief medical officer (CMO) early morning, saying that his office would be sending samples by afternoon. We used to wait for the samples, and they would reach us at varied times, from 6.00 p.m. to 10.00 p.m. at times. The lab work used to start after the samples were received. Sometimes, it used to so happen that the commissioner's office informed that a sample was on its way from a particular district and needed to be tested that day itself. The staff in the BSL-2 lab was made to wait in their PPE suits to process those samples. This was to save the PPE kits as there was a shortage of kits.

The number of samples increased by the day, and the samples mostly tested negative. On the evening of 30 March, one sample of a post-mortem case showed positive results in the screening assay. The sample was transported immediately to KGMU, Lucknow, for confirmation of the results. This was the first laboratory-confirmed case of COVID-19 and also the first death associated with COVID-19 in the eastern part of Uttar Pradesh.

The first positive detection brought a sense of fear among the staff who was involved in the testing of that sample. The fear subsided after the staff members tested negative on the fifth and the tenth day, following exposure.

Most often, work used to start in the evening (7.00–9.00 p.m.) and it extended up to 4.00–5.00 a.m. Staff members used to leave for their homes after having a bath late at night. Me and my colleagues and the data entry operator, would stay back to finish reporting and dispatching reports. Due to lockdown restrictions, the official vehicle driver was asked to drop us home early morning, which, after a few days, was annoying to the driver. Hence, we scientists decided to get our bicycles and ride them back home early in morning!

Sometimes, we were also stopped by the police for checking and most often they used to request us to help them to get their samples tested after getting to know we worked in the COVID-19 lab! This morning bicycle ride was indeed comforting, as the roads were empty and the air was fresh. But the pleasurable rides were ruined by the street dogs, who chased us while we pedalled away furiously to avoid being bitten by them. They, of course, did not know that we were busy saving the nation from a pandemic!

4: THE GAME CHANGER

1. Gupta, Nivedita et al., 'Laboratory Preparedness for SARS-Cov-2 Testing in India: Harnessing a Network of Virus Research & Diagnostic Laboratories', *Indian Journal of Medical Research*, Vol. 151, No. 2 & 3, February–March 2020, pp. 216–225. DOI: 10.4103/ijmr.IJMR_594_20.

2. 'How India Scaled Up Its Laboratory Testing Capacity for COVID19', World Health Organization News, 16 August 2020, https://www.who.int/india/news/feature-stories/detail/how-india-scaled-up-its-laboratory-testing-capacity-for-covid19.

3. 'Revised Guidelines for TrueNat Testing for COVID-19', Indian Council of Medical Research, 24 September 2020.

4. Gupta, Nivedita et al., 'Innovative Point-Of-Care Molecular

Diagnostic Test For COVID-19 In India', The Lancet Microbe, Vol. 1, No. 7, November 2020, https://doi.org/10.1016/S2666-5247(20)30164-6.

5. 'Newer Additional Strategies for COVID-19 Testing', Indian Council of Medical Research, 23 June 2020.

5: WHY RESEARCH MATTERS

1. Dovih, Pilot et al., 'Filovirus-Reactive Antibodies in Humans and Bats in Northeast India Imply Zoonotic Spillover', *PLoS Neglected Tropical Diseases*, Vol. 13, No. 10, October 2019. DOI: https://doi.org/10.1371/journal.pntd.0007733.

2. Yadav, Pragya D. et al., 'Detection of Corona Viruses in Pteropus & Rousettus Species of Bats from Different States of India', *Indian Journal of Medical Research*, Vol. 151, No. 2 & 3, pp.226–235. DOI: 10.4103/ijmr.IJMR_795_20.

3. Adapted from 'The Story of the PLACID Trial—A Democratisation of Research', *theBMJopinion*, 2 November 2020, https://blogs.bmj.com/bmj/2020/11/02/the-story-of-the-placid-trial-a-democratization-of-research/.

4. Agarwal, Anup et al., 'Convalescent Plasma in the Management of Moderate COVID-19 in Adults in India: Open Label Phase II Multicenter Randomized Controlled Trial (Placid Trial)', *British Medical Journal*, Vol. 22, October 2020. DOI: 10.1136/bmj.m3939.

5. 'WHO COVID-19 Solidarity Therapeutics Trial', WHO, https://www.who.int/emergencies/diseases/novel-coronavirus-2019/global-research-on-novel-coronavirus-2019-ncov/solidarity-clinical-trial-for-covid-19-treatments.

6. Pan, Hongchao et al., 'Repurposed Antiviral Drugs for COVID-19—Interim WHO Solidarity Trial Results', *New England Journal of Medicine*, Vol. 384, No. 6, February 2020, pp. 497–511. DOI: 10.1056/NEJMoa2023184.

7. Dr Sheela Godbole from ICMR-NARI remembers,

    > India's Solidarity treatment trial was initiated by the ICMR in a very short time at 26 trial sites, amidst a lot of challenges, when the country was in a state of intense lockdown. At that time, it was difficult to cross state borders and we would not have been able to shift the study drugs to trial sites without the intervention of Prof. Bhargava. One letter from him acted like magic and we could quickly shift the drugs under controlled conditions all over India from Pune,
    >
    > There was a time when the only stock of Remdesivir in India was with the trial team. Although the drug was still investigational, many people in desperation requested its use on compassionate grounds. While I could understand their sentiment, the use was against the trial principles. Prof. Bhargava stood by us when we were under severe pressure to use the drug. He said, 'Follow the science and stand by scientific principles'.

8. Dr Rajni Kant from ICMR-RMRC, Gorakhpur recollects an incident,

9 April 2021 was the last day of my week-long tour of Gorakhpur and I was getting ready to return to Delhi. Early in the morning I received a WhatsApp message from one of my colleagues, stating that he was not feeling well since last evening, he got tested and was positive for COVID-19. He advised that those who were in contact should also get tested. Since the situation was not that bad at that point in time, we were having regular meetings, although we followed social distancing and other norms.

It had been a busy week and we were interacting with many of the staff members, including scientists, to discuss various issues and future programmes. We had organized a swachhta day, inviting a renowned cyclist and environmentalist two days ago. To my utter surprise, when the results of testing were disclosed, out of 60 staff members that were tested, 35 were positive. I had also given my sample, but fortunately I was negative.

I was deeply tense and scared as all those who were around me throughout the week were Covid positive. Even the drivers who used to take me from the guest house daily and who picked and dropped me at the airport, as well as my personal secretary and many of the scientists and administrative staff, had tested positive. I tried to isolate myself for a week and took utmost care, wearing mask while at home. I got myself retested after a week. As an immediate measure, all those who had tested

171

positive were asked to rest at home, start treatment and follow other protocols.

A few days later, the condition of one of the colleagues deteriorated and he was admitted in the ICU. He became critical in successive days with severe depletion in oxygen saturation and lung infection. But after initial hiccups, and with the grace of God, he began responding to treatment and recovered. However, later, the health condition of two others also worsened, and despite all medical interventions, they could not be saved. One lost his life two months after recovery, perhaps due to post-Covid complications. We were heart-broken. Either the two doses of Covaxin taken earlier, coupled with Covid appropriate behaviour saved me, or it was the hand of God.

9. Dr Debjit Chakraborty from ICMR- NICED, Kolkata shares his experience,

The hard work continues post my personal battle with Covid. It is needless to mention that the healthcare professionals who have recovered from the disease are the armed soldiers of the society who are fighting the virus from the front. While access to healthcare has always been a challenge for the rural communities in a country like ours, the pandemic has aggravated the problem manifold. It is of utmost importance that the healthcare providers, who are also Covid survivors, make efforts to reach out to the farthest and the remotest corners of the country to assess the spread of the disease and take measures accordingly.

I was visiting one such rural area in West Bengal in the East Medinipur district as a part of the second round of the ICMR National COVID-19 sero-surveillance, where the lonely footbridge over river Kangsabati had been destroyed due to Amphan (the 2020 cyclone), leading to the total collapse of connectivity between the villages on one side and the primary health-care facilities on the other.

So, we had to cross the river using a small wooden boat (a 'Dingi' in Bengali) that could bear the load of a maximum of three people at a time. Consequently, the three of us in the survey team sat precariously on the rain-drenched edge of the boat and tried to hold onto each other in the face of unruly tides of the river on a cloudy monsoon afternoon. There was a good chance that the boat would topple and we would all drown. But we stayed afloat, to fight the bigger battle of restoring health and happiness in the society.

Humans need to act as a bridge between darkness and light, between despair and hope, between death and life. I am proud of all the Covid warriors.

10. Dr Debdutta Bhattacharya from ICMR-RMRC, Bhubaneswar recollects,

In view of the increase in cases in late March, our director general decided to use the high-throughput Cobas machines installed in the country, for diagnosis of SARS-CoV-2 infections. In continuation with this, the government of Odisha, through the Odisha Industrial Infrastructure Development Corporation (IDCO), made infrastructural modification for laboratory space to develop the BSL-2 plus facility required for testing. A vendor was selected to developing BSL-2 plus facility by the end of March 2020.

Thereafter, one fine Sunday morning of 5 April 2020, I got a call from my director. 'We need to make the BSL-2 plus facility for Cobas Laboratory functional in 2–4 days.' I went numb, wondering how that was possible. Subsequently we got a call from the ICMR higher authorities. 'Beta, let us know what you require, we will give all possible support, but get the materials of laboratory infrastructure and HR lifted from the designated vendor and HR support from Chennai.'

We called the vendor stationed in Chennai, and with lot of 'illa' (no) and 'seri' (yes), we could finally convince them to board the IAF AN 32 from Chennai on 5 April 2020, along with laboratory panels and biosafety cabinet weighing about 3,500 kilograms, and 19 engineers. At 1.00 a.m., along with the Odisha State Medical Corporation official and our office drivers, we reached the cargo section of Bhubaneswar airport airstrip. Two flights with Air Force officers, one a lady pilot, handed over the materials and completed the formalities. While leaving, they said, 'Sir, you guys are doing a wonderful job. The entire country is looking up to you all.' I replied back with 'Jai Hind!'

6: AN INDIAN VACCINE: FROM DREAM TO ROLL-OUT

1. Riedel, Stefan, 'Edward Jenner and the History of Smallpox and Vaccination', *Baylor University Medical Center Proceedings*, Vol. 18, No. 1, January 2005, pp. 21–25. DOI: 10.1080/08998280.2005.11928028.

The author writes that,'For many years, he had heard the tales that dairymaids were protected from smallpox naturally after having suffered from cowpox. Pondering this, Jenner concluded that cowpox not only protected against smallpox but also could be transmitted from one person to another as a deliberate mechanism of protection. In May 1796, Edward Jenner found a young dairymaid, Sarah Nelms, who had fresh cowpox lesions on her hands and arms. On May 14, 1796, using matter from Nelms' lesions, he inoculated an 8-year-old boy, James Phipps. Subsequently, the boy developed mild fever and discomfort in the axillae. Nine days after the procedure he felt cold and had lost his appetite, but on the next day he was much better. In July 1796, Jenner inoculated the boy again, this time with matter from a fresh smallpox lesion. No disease developed, and Jenner concluded that protection was complete.'

2. Roos, Dave, 'How a New Vaccine Was Developed in Record Time in the 1960s', *History*, 22 June 2020, https://www. history.com/news/mumps-vaccine-world-war-ii. The author narrates the interesting incident about mumps vaccine, 'At 1 a.m. on March 21, 1963, a five-year-old girl in Philadelphia woke her father, Dr. Maurice Hilleman, complaining of a sore throat. Hilleman, a prickly genius working at Merck, immediately diagnosed her with a case of the mumps, a generally harmless childhood illness for which there was no treatment, and sent her back to bed.

But Hilleman couldn't go back to sleep—he had an idea. Another research lab had just licensed a measles vaccine based on a new technique for growing weakened forms of a live virus in chicken embryos. Maybe he could do the same thing for mumps. Hilleman rushed to Merck for sampling supplies, came back and swabbed his daughter's throat, then drove the viral culture back to the lab.

The mumps vaccine Hilleman developed in 1967 from that late-night inspiration is still in use as part of the combination measles, mumps and rubella (MMR) vaccine given to infants the world over. In the United States alone, mumps used to infect 186,000 kids a year in the 1960s. Today, thanks to the vaccine, there are fewer than 1,000 mumps infections annually.

Perhaps the most charming part of Hilleman's mumps vaccine story is that he named the strain of mumps virus used to make the vaccine after his young daughter, Jeryl

Lynn. The same Jeryl Lynn strain is still used in mumps vaccine production today.'

3. https://www.bharatbiotech.com/revacb_mcf.html.

4. 'COVID-19 Vaccine Tracker and Landscape', World Health Organization, 7 September 2021, https://www.who.int/publications/m/item/draft-landscape-of-covid-19-candidate-vaccines.

5. Pardi, Nobert et al., 'mRNA vaccines—a new era in vaccinology', *Nature Reviews Drug Discovery*, Vol. 17, pp. 261–279, https://doi.org/10.1038/nrd.2017.243.

6. Ganneru, Brunda et al., 'Th1 Skewed Immune Response of Whole Virion Inactivated SARS-Cov- 2 Vaccine and Its Safety Evaluation', *iScience*, Vol. 24, No. 4, April 2021, https://doi.org/10.1016/j.isci.2021.102298.

7. Mohandas, Sreelekshmy et al., 'Immunogenicity and Protective Efficacy of BBV152, Whole Virion Inactivated SARS-Cov-2 Vaccine Candidates in the Syrian Hamster Model', *iScience*, Vol. 24, No. 2, February 2021, pp. 1–27, https://doi.org/10.1016/j.isci.2021.102054.

8. Dr Pragya Yadav from ICMR-NIV takes a look back on the ordeal of arranging sufficient number of animals required for the small animal study,

> We enquired for hamsters in nearby institutes and animal facilities in Maharashtra, but were not available. When Director, ICMR-NIN, Hyderabad, Dr Hemlata, was contacted, she readily agreed to provide her support to this noble cause. The staff of ICMR-NIN brought the animals by road to Pune

amid the COVID-19 imposed restrictions, taking utmost biosafety precautions.

We felt delight seeing those animals, and our veterinary team took the best care of these creatures who will tell us if the vaccine is good. Dr Sreelekshmy Mohandas and rest of team completed this hamster study timely.

9. Going back in time, Dr Pragya Yadav from ICMR-NIV, Pune remembers,

> A team including Dr M.D. Gokhale and Dr Dilip Patil from ICMR-NIV went to the areas in Pune Forest Division with the Forest Department staff. The team could not find any Rhesus macaque in that belt. Again, permission was sought for the Nanded region from PCCF, Maharashtra. With much difficulty, we managed to trace a professional monkey catcher from Miraj. But during the last minute, he backed off, citing reasons of shortage of staff and vehicle due to COVID-19. The team travelled to Nanded and located a few areas where Rhesus macaques are present. With the help of the Forest Department and a local professional monkey catcher, the team managed to trap a few macaques. Due to less number of animals in that area, permission was sought from PCCF, Maharashtra to capture required animals from Nagpur region. The team along with the catcher travelled to Nagpur for trapping monkeys. Due

to the scarcity in food availability in the urban dwellings, macaques migrated to deep forests making it a tough time for the team. Finally, the team was able to trap the sufficient number of macaques after spending around twenty days in the field. Arranging transport back was another challenge. Forest department helped in the arranging the transport of the animals.

10. Dr Pragya Yadav from ICMR-NIV, Pune remembers,

On being requested for team support, the Commandant, Army Institute of Cardio-Thoracic Sciences (AICTS), Pune said that soldiers fought against enemies in war, whenever the motherland gave a call. This too was a war, he added, and extended his institute's full support. The team members were trained to work inside the containment laboratory, which involved risks like animal handling, working with sharps, etc. They did practise with Dr Sanjay Kumar in a timed manner to complete each activity in harmony. There were days when the team worked in the containment facility for really long hours. No laboratory accidents or incidents were recorded during the period, indicating the alertness of the staff even under tiring and stressful work hours. From other departments, Dr Basavaj Mathapti and Dr Himanshu Kaushal joined us to complete the task.

11. Yadav, Pragya D. et al., 'Immunogenicity and Protective Efficacy of Inactivated SARS-Cov-2 Vaccine Candidate, BBV152 in Rhesus Macaques', *Nature Communications*, Vol. 12, No. 1, March 2021, pp. 1–11, https://doi.org/10.1038/s41467-021-21639-w.

7: THE MOMENT OF TRUTH

1. Ella, Raches et al., 'Safety And Immunogenicity of an Inactivated SARS-Cov-2 Vaccine, BBV152: A Double-Blind, Randomised, Phase 1 Trial', *The Lancet Infectious Diseases*, Vol. 21, No. 5, January 2021, pp. 637–646, https://doi.org/10.1016/S1473-3099(20)30942-7.

2. Ella, Raches, et al., 'Safety and Immunogenicity of an Inactivated SARS-Cov-2 Vaccine, BBV152: Interim Results from a Double-Blind, Randomised, Multicentre, Phase 2 Trial, and 3-Month Follow-Up of a Double-Blind, Randomised Phase 1 Trial', *The Lancet Infectious Diseases*, Vol. 21, No. 7, March 2021, pp. 950–961. DOI: 10.1016/S1473-3099(21)00070-0.

3. Ghose, Tia, 'What Are Antibodies?', *Livescience*, 17 July 2020, https://www.livescience.com/antibodies.html.

4. 'Types of Antibodies', MBL Life Sciences, https://ruo.mbl.co.jp/bio/e/support/method/antibody-role.html.

5. Ella, Raches et al., 'Efficacy, Safety, and Lot to Lot Immunogenicity of an Inactivated SARS-Cov-2 Vaccine 2 (BBV152): A, Double-Blind, Randomised, Controlled Phase 3 Trial', *medRxiv*, July 2021, https://www.medrxiv.org/content/10.1101/2021.06.30.21259439v1.

6. Yadav, Pragya D. et al., 'Isolation and Characterization of the New SARS-Cov-2 Variant in Travellers from the United Kingdom to India: VUI-202012/01 of the B.1.1.7 Lineage', *Journal of Travel Medicine*, Vol. 28, No. 2, March 2021. DOI: 10.1093/jtm/taab009.

7. Rostad, Christina A and Anderson Evan J, 'Optimism and Caution for an Inactivated COVID-19 Vaccine', *Lancet Infectious Disease*, Vol. 21, No. 5, May 2021, pp. 581–582. DOI: 10.1016/S1473-3099(20)30988-9.

8. Li, Jing-Xin and Zhu, Feng-Cai, 'Adjuvantation Helps to Optimise COVID-19 Vaccine Candidate', *Lancet Infectious Diseases*, Vol. 21, No. 7, March 2021, pp. 891–893. doi: 10.1016/S1473-3099(21)00094-3; The authors have highlighted that the inactivated whole-virus vaccine platform is the most well-established manufacturing platform for vaccine production, and aluminium salts are the most commonly used adjuvants used in human vaccines. Thus, an alum-adjuvanted whole-virion inactivated vaccine is a logical step in the development of a COVID-19 vaccine.

9. 'Virus Neutralization', *Encyclopedia of Virology Third Edition*, Elsevier, 2008. https://www.sciencedirect.com/topics/medicine-and-dentistry/virus-neutralization.

10. Yadav, Pragya D. et al., 'Isolation and Characterization of the New SARS-Cov-2 Variant in Travellers from the United Kingdom to India: VUI-202012/01 of the B.1.1.7 Lineage', *Journal of Travel Medicine*, Vol. 28, No. 2, March 2021. DOI: 10.1093/jtm/taab009.

11. 'Tracking   SARS-CoV-2   Variants',   World   Health

Organization, https://www.who.int/en/activities/tracking-SARS-CoV-2-variants/.

12. Yadav, Pragya D. et al., 'Neutralization of Beta and Delta Variant with Sera of COVID-19 Recovered Cases and Vaccines of Inactivated COVID-19 Vaccine BBV152/COVAXIN', *Journal of Travel Medicine*; Vol. 28, No. 5, July 2021, pp. 1–3. DOI: 10.1093/jtm/taab104.

13. Sapkal, Gajanan et al., 'Inactivated COVID-19 Vaccine BBV152/COVAXIN Effectively Neutralizes Recently Emerged B.1.1.7 Variant of SARS-Cov-2', *Journal of Travel Medicine*, Vol. 28, No. 4, May 2021, pp. 1–10. DOI: 10.1093/jtm/taab051.

14. Sapkal, Gajanan et al., 'Neutralization of B.1.1.28 P2 Variant with Sera of Natural SARS-Cov-2 Infection and Recipients of Inactivated COVID-19 Vaccine Covaxin', *Journal of Travel Medicine*. Vol. 28, No. 4, May 2021. DOI: 10.1093/jtm/taab077.

15. Gupta, Indrani and Baru, Rama, 'Economics & Ethics of the COVID-19 Vaccine: How Prepared Are We?' *Indian Journal of Medical Research*, Vol. 152, No. 1 & 2, 2020, pp. 153–155. doi: 10.4103/ijmr.IJMR_3581_20.

16. Dinda, Amit K. et al., 'Revisiting Regulatory Framework in India for Accelerated Vaccine Development in Pandemics with an Evidence-Based Fast-Tracking Strategy', *Indian Journal of Medical Research*, Vol. 152, No. 1 & 2, 2020, pp. 156–163. doi: 10.4103/ijmr.IJMR_3640_20.

17. 'Restricted Use of COVAXIN™ under Clinical Trial Mode', Ministry of Health and Family Welfare, 11 January 2021.

8: RISE OF A VACCINE SUPERPOWER

1. Gross, C.P. and Sepkowitz, K.A., 'The Myth of the Medical Breakthrough: Smallpox, Vaccination, and Jenner Reconsidered', *International Journal of Infectious Disease*, Vol. 3, No. 1, July–September 1998, pp. 54–60. DOI: 10.1016/s1201-9712(98)90096-0.

   The author records the earliest proof of variolation, 'Lady Mary Wortley Montagu (1689-1762) lived in Turkey with her husband, the ambassador Edward Wortley Montagu.' It was there that Lady Montagu first witnessed inoculation, in 1716, and subsequently had her son inoculated. It is thought that her dedication to preventing the disease grew from the fact that her own once beautiful face had been disfigured by smallpox. Two years later, having returned to England, Lady Montagu had her daughter inoculated during a smallpox epidemic, under the scrutiny of the Royal Society's Physicians.

   The inoculation was considered successful when the child developed a limited number of lesions and did not contract overwhelming disease.'

2. Bennett, C.H. and Bannerman, W.B. 'Inoculation of an Entire Community with Haffkine's Plague Vaccine', *The Indian Medical Gazette*, Vol. 34 No. 6, June 1899, pp. 192–193.

   The author summarizes the results of Plague vaccination, 'The numbers attacked in the regiment kept pace exactly with the severity of the epidemic in the neighbouring town, rising and declining with it. We have seen how heavily the regiment suffered during the first epidemic, so their escape at this time requires explanation. The only measures taken by the authorities were placing the cantonment and city "out of bounds " for the troops after 4th July, and the disinfection of the few huts that became infected. Both these measures had been taken in the first outbreak and had proved totally inadequate. How then did the regiment escape during the second outbreak ? The men of the regiment were so satisfied with the effect produced by the first inoculation, that they made no objection to being reinoculated in August, and this operation was so thoroughly performed that practically no one in the lines were left unprotected.'

3. *The Indian Empire: A Brief Description of the Chief Features of India and Its Medical and Sanitary Problems*, Thacker's Directories, 1927, p. 298.

4. 'Indian Pharmaceutical Industry Report', Indian Brand Equity Foundation, July 2021, https://www.ibef.org/industry/pharmaceutical-india.aspx.

5. 'Indian Pharmaceuticals—a Formula for Success', *Invest India*, https://www.investindia.gov.in/sector/pharmaceuticals.

6. 'Value of Indian Pharmaceutical Exports from Financial year 2012 to 2021', *statista*, https://www.statista.com/statistics/1038136/india-value-of-pharmaceutical-exports/#:~:text=India%20is%20the%20world's%20largest,America%20had%20the%20largest%20share.

7. 'Indian Pharmaceuticals—a Formula for Success', *Invest India*, https://www.investindia.gov.in/sector/pharmaceuticals.

8. Mandal, Sandip et al., 'India's Pragmatic Vaccination Strategy against COVID-19: A Mathematical Modelling-Based Analysis', *BMJ Open*, Vo. 11, No. 7, July 2021. DOI: 10.1136/bmjopen-2021-048874.

9. Dr Sanghamitra Pati from ICMR-RMRC, Bhubaneswar shares an interesting incident,

> My memorable moment dates back to the initial weeks of the first national lockdown. It must have been late, past midnight. It was usual for all of us at the centre to work till late at night, ours being the only lead laboratory for RT-PCR testing. I was returning from my centre after attending a video conferencing meeting followed by the routine discussion on laboratory issues with my colleagues. Apart from a few distantly beeping ambulances and patrolling vans, the road looked deserted with not a single soul outside. Such unusual silent nights were our regular companion while we returned from the lab those days.
>
> Suddenly, at the second main square, the vehicle halted with a jolt, as someone signalled us to stop. Moving a little closer, I found a traffic person on night duty. It took me a few seconds to get a feel of the situation. A wave of mixed feelings of confusion and apprehension swept over me. As a knee-jerk reaction, I started scrambling for my ID card in frenzy, forgetting that it was around my neck. To be honest, I was feeling a little irked too.

Does n't the traffic person know that we are working in a COVID testing lab? After all, we had got the due transport pass from the authority, visibly fixed on the front-glass pane of the vehicle. Being a traffic guy, he should have noticed that!

Then I thought, maybe he was doing his duty. After all, it was past midnight, and apart from police patrol and ambulance I was the sole non-such vehicle rider, so he had every reason to be inquisitive.

I looked at him quizzically through the open window, holding the ID card as proof of evidence, hoping sincerely that he would decipher the gesture from my masked face from a distance. However, the he came walking towards the window, and maintaining a guarded social distance greeted me. He said, 'Madam, please excuse me. I did not want to distract you from your duty. We all are well aware of the hard work that your centre and your team are doing for the people in such crisis moments. We all are grateful to you. I had always wanted to convey my sentiments to you personally, but was not getting a chance. Tonight, thankfully, I am on duty here, and when I saw your vehicle with the ICMR-RMRC Bhubaneswar sticker, I could not resist myself from stopping you for a second. This is just to compliment you and salute your team for all the hard work you are doing for all of us and the state and the country.

From all my colleagues, I wish to convey our best wishes to your team of corona warriors. We are with you and hopeful that with your support the country can evict this corona.'

For a second, I was completely taken aback. To be candid, I was not expecting this serendipitous laurel at midnight from a traffic controller, who is always busy with streamlining the unruly vehicles.

My eyes welled with tears. It was truly an overwhelming moment. My spontaneous response was, 'Brother, you and your fraternity are also doing an equally great job during these challenging times, day and night, towards containing this unknown virus. Each one of us is a corona warrior. Fighting with corona is a team marathon, and requires your and our relentless efforts, towards this end. When we all have united for the unified cause, we can win the war.'

He nodded and I could see his eyes sparkling with a ray of hope and confidence, infused with tears of pride and patriotism. I thanked him with folded hands. Though brief, with minimal verbal exchange, this interlude at midnight weaved a thread of connectedness of commitment to curb the pandemic. The spirit of 'together we can win', reverberated strongly amidst the silent night. We all had to rise to the occasion, and we did.

I always used to feel proud of the ICMR, but being a part of the COVID-19 war armamentarium, was immensely overpowering, and poignantly momentous for me, as I counted my blessings. How many of us get an opportunity to serve at such critical junctures in a war mode for our own motherland, society and people? It added value and a meaningful purpose to our profession. Today too, while reminiscing those small yet energy-rich moments in the COVID-19 chronicle, I feel electrified. Let this dedication and passion of doing for the country and with the country remain our eternal professional virtue. Vande Mataram!

10. Panda, Samiran, 'Talking Vaccine Hesitancy', *The Hindu*, 21 April 2021, https://www.thehindu.com/opinion/op-ed/tackling-vaccine-hesitancy/article34369937.ece.

11. Perappadan, Bindu S. 'We Are Dealing with a Virus which Is Easily Transmissible and Leaves a Devastating Effect, Says ICMR Scientist', *The Hindu*, 15 January 2021, https://www.thehindu.com/news/national/we-are-dealing-with-a-virus-which-is-easily-transmissible-and-leaves-a-devastating-effect-says-icmr-scientist/article33580874.ece.

12. Panda, Samiran et al. 'Face Mask an Essential Armour in the Fight of India Against COVID-19', *Indian Journal of Medical Research*, Vol. 153, No. 1, March 2021, pp. 233–37, https://www.ijmr.org.in/text.asp?2021/153/1/233/308604.

13. Anand, Tanu et al. 'Reopening of Schools during COVID-19 Pandemic: A Persistent Dilemma', *Indian Journal of Medical Research*, Vol. 153, May–June 2021, pp. 572–76. DOI: 10.4103/ijmr.ijmr_2805_21.

14. Mandal, Sandeep et al. 'Responsible Travel to and within India during the COVID-19 Pandemic', *Journal of Travel Medicine*, September 2021. DOI: 10.1093/jtm/taab147.

INDEX

Index